THE DAKOTA DIET

Health Secrets from the Great Plains

Kevin Weiland, M.D., FACP

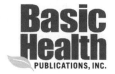

Basic Health
PUBLICATIONS, INC.

The information contained in this book is based upon the research and personal and professional experiences of the author. It is not intended as a substitute for consulting with your physician or other healthcare provider. Any attempt to diagnose and treat an illness should be done under the direction of a healthcare professional.

The publisher does not advocate the use of any particular healthcare protocol but believes the information in this book should be available to the public. The publisher and author are not responsible for any adverse effects or consequences resulting from the use of the suggestions, preparations, or procedures discussed in this book. Should the reader have any questions concerning the appropriateness of any procedures or preparation mentioned, the author and the publisher strongly suggest consulting a professional healthcare advisor.

Basic Health Publications, Inc.
28812 Top of the World Drive
Laguna Beach, CA 92651
949-715-7327 • www.basichealthpub.com

Library of Congress Cataloging-in-Publication Data
Weiland, Kevin
    The Dakota diet : health secrets from the Great Plains / Kevin Weiland.
        p. cm.
    Includes bibliographical references and index.
    ISBN 978-1-59120-205-9
1. Omega-3 fatty acids—Health aspects. 2. Diet. 3. Essential fatty acids
in human nutrition. 4. Health. I. Title.

    QP752.O44W4557   2007
    612.3'97—dc22

                                          2007003192

Editor: John Anderson
Typesetting/Book design: Gary A. Rosenberg
Cover design: Mike Stromberg

Printed in the United States of America

10   9   8   7   6   5   4   3   2   1

Contents

This book is dedicated to
Joseph John,
Josie Rose,
John Paul,
and Annie Laurie

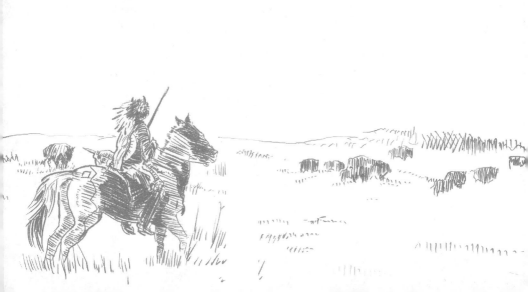

Acknowledgments

First and foremost, I would like to thank the *Rapid City Journal* and their editorial staff for allowing me to write a monthly preventative medicine column. In doing so, I have learned to better communicate with my patients and have gained a tremendous amount of respect for the journalistic profession. Thanks to my veteran nurse Gaile Eckert, for taking me under her wing and guiding me to a successful primary care practice. Her skill and efficiency as a nurse allowed me to provide the best care to my patients and find enough time to enjoy my family and write this book.

A special thanks to Kenny and Linnea Putnam and Kassi Jolley of Image Up for their creative skills as well as making sure the manuscript was ready for the publisher. I'd like to thank Charlie Abourezk and Dr. Brett Lawlor for reviewing early versions and providing invaluable insight when needed. Thanks also to Ruth Whitcher for her ongoing advice and editing throughout the years.

I am deeply grateful to author and physician, Dr. Stephen T. Sinatra, for introducing me to the publisher of Basic Health and for writing a foreword to this book.

Thanks to Norman Goldfind of Basic Health Publications for taking the time to meet with me in order to review my manuscript and deciding to take me on as a first-time author. I hope we can do this again—real soon. And to my editor, John Anderson, who helped make the book readable and patiently worked with me while I continued to write as well as practice medicine full time.

Thanks to Vince Green and Mark Johnson for their encouragement and advice in getting the book published and to Holly Lemay for her pioneering work with school nutrition and physical education in our community. Thanks also to Charles McClain.

This book could never have been produced without the talents and recipes of the contributing chefs. South Dakota's own chef Virginia Koster of public radio's "Prairie Gourmet," chef Sanaa Abourezk of Sanaa's Restaurant, and Jill McGuire (our buffalo queen).

Thanks to Kibbe Conti for helping guide my patients to healthier living through nutrition as well as for her nutritional advice and support for this book. A special thanks to the Rapid City Regional Hospital dietary department for their help with nutritional analysis.

Most of all, I want to thank my wife, Dr. Laurie Weisensee, a physician in her own right and the mother of our three children, Laurie's passion for knowledge on nutrition gave me inspiration and I thank her for the support, time, and invaluable input. And her passion for buffalo will someday (I am sure) land her the ranch she so truly deserves.

Foreword

by Stephen T. Sinatra, M.D.

When Dr. Weiland requested that I write a Foreword to this book, I was quite intrigued by both his topic and his title, *The Dakota Diet*. As a bit of a Civil War buff, I must confess that the state of Dakota conjures up images of open plains and grazing buffalo for me—life the way it used to be. I was equally impressed that the content is consistent with the health advice I dole out to subscribers of my newsletter, *Heart, Health and Nutrition*. Dr. Weiland describes how to follow a healthy, non-inflammatory, non–insulin provoking eating plan, which means selecting health-promoting foods including buffalo, nuts, fruits, vegetables, legumes, flaxseeds, healthy fish, and more.

If you choose to follow the advice in this book, you'll slash your risk of having to deal with health concerns like diabetes, high blood pressure, heart disease, and cancer. And while I may not endorse a couple of details—like the use of canola oil, artificial sweeteners, and statin drugs to drop cholesterol in folks without heart disease—I am in whole-hearted agreement with Dr. Weiland's food and dietary recommendations. The most important feature that sets this "diet book" apart from all others is its recognition of the importance of selecting grass-fed buffalo (also known as bison) as a primary meat choice.

One of the reasons a seasoned cardiologist like me chooses and recommends grass-fed buffalo is that it's part of a healthy eating plan to avoid problems like heart disease. Grass-fed bison also contains up to 500% more conjugated linoleic acid (CLA) than beef fed on conventional grain diets, and the advantages of CLA are numerous. CLA perks include lowering LDL ("bad") cholesterol levels in the blood, normalizing blood glucose, inducing a decrease in body fat, and enhancing immune system function. CLA also helps thwart allergies and asthma. Buffalo is very lean and has only a fraction of the fat that you'll find in beef, pork, or even chicken. And bison grazing on a purely grass diet produce a lean beef that's essentially 95% fat free. Not only is their meat lower in calories, it's also higher in iron and essential fatty acids than conventional beef.

And the best part of eating 100% grass-fed bison is that you won't be getting a product that's been developed according to guidelines set up by the U.S. beef industry. Most of the meat we eat is no longer in the natural form our forefathers put on the table. We eat meats from animals fed a grain diet. The trouble is that cattle aren't designed to eat grains just because that's what is convenient to farmers. They were meant to be grazing in green fields, like their ancestors. All that grass, and all that walking to find it, meant lean meat for our survival in generations past.

Another problem is that in order to harvest more grain to feed those animals, non-organic farmers often rely on fertilizers, pesticides, and herbicides. In addition to the quality of the feed, the beef industry has created "super cattle," animals "pumped up" with antibiotics and hormones so they produce more milk and tip the scales in the marketplace. This point was unhappily brought home to me recently as I lectured to an audience local to my home in Connecticut. I asked if there were any dairy farmers in the audience. One woman raised her hand. When I asked her whether or not she gave hormones to her cattle, her response was that she was "not allowed to say." Not allowed to say? Scary, isn't it?

So, the meat products on our dinner tables hardly resemble the grass-fed meat of decades ago. And while absolute fat content is an issue, it's what is in that fat that's the real problem. Pesticides, herbicides, hormones, and antibiotics concentrate themselves in fatty tissues—the same fat that's on that steak you love to splurge on! Consuming grain-fed commercial beef means that a significant toxic load is dumped into your body. Your safest bet is to consume buffalo or bison.

In an ideal world, we would all eat only free-range beef and chicken or fresh-caught fish from non-polluted waters, like wild Alaskan salmon (never farm-raised fish, like salmon, as their flesh is pinkened with dye pellets and their waters are often contaminated). We'd eliminate, or at least avoid, produce that's been exposed to fertilizers, pesticides, and herbicides. We would look for the word "organic" on our food selections as much is possible. However, living up to this ideal is difficult, if not impossible, in our fast-paced world.

So, I truly appreciate the contribution that Dr. Weiland has made in developing the Dakota Diet. He proposes that we all select diets rich in omega-3 essential fatty acids and the vital phytonutrients found in other equally health-promoting foods. *The Dakota Diet* is based on solid scientific principles, and this book offers a comprehensive bibliography.

On a personal note, eating food the way nature intended it to be is not just important for your own health, it's also key to supporting our environment and animal welfare as well. That also means eating fruits, vegetables, grains, and meats in season, and being mindful of how they are brought to your home. Remember, the old adage "you are what you eat." When you make the decision to eat "Dakota style," you'll also be supporting our agrarian society and farmers who want to do the right thing. Supporting our farmland and our environment can make you feel more connected with your food while taking an important step in your quest for optimum health.

—Stephen T. Sinatra, M.D., F.A.C.C., C.N.S.
Author of *Reverse Heart Disease Now* (Wiley, 2007)
and *The Sinatra Solution* (Basic Health, 2007)

Foreword

by Tom Daschle

One of the great myths of America is that we have the best health care system in the world. We do have some extraordinary clinics and hospitals and many health providers who are among the world's best. But for the majority of Americans who are not fortunate enough to access one of these facilities, the story is vastly different. For them, because of increasingly serious problems in our system relating to cost, access and quality, their circumstances are much different. As a result, today the United States ranks 35th in life expectancy in the world and only 41st in infant mortality. When it comes to our nation's health care system, in reality we have what some have called "islands of excellence in a sea of mediocrity."

To make matters worse, we now pay $6,700 annually per capita in premiums, taxes and out-of-pocket expenses. That is at least 40% more than the next most expensive country. Our national health costs will soon exceed $2 trillion, comprising nearly 20% of our entire economy. And the costs continue to rise exponentially. In just the last five years, costs have risen by nearly 100%.

In spite of these costs, or more accurately, in part because of them, 47 million Americans have no health insurance. Over a half million people are added to the roles of the uninsured in our country every year. As they become ill and need care, they oftentimes forgo treatment or attempt to access our system in its most expensive form, the emergency room.

No one is immune from the problems of our broken health care system. Even if one has health insurance and can afford to pay the exorbitant costs today, the American system can even be dangerous. An estimated 300 million mistakes are made every year and over 100,000 deaths occur as a result of those mistakes or because many have little or no access to health care.

Perhaps the biggest reason for medical errors is the health care system's reliance on an administrative system that is largely paper driven. That is particularly ironic, given the health industry's increasing reliance on technology.

The United States badly needs comprehensive health care reform. It is my hope that we will soon see the day when a new system can be created.

One of the most important characteristics of any good health care system is a recognition and implementation of wellness promotion, prevention and effective primary care. It is already emphasized in most industrialized as well as developing countries in the world. It is the most cost effective health care available today, just as it has been for centuries.

But unfortunately, over my lifetime, the American health care system has moved away from the most basic and cost effective forms of health care delivery. As a result, some experts now call obesity in America a pandemic. Statistically, my grandchildren's generation may have an even shorter life expectancy than that of my generation in part because of this growing health crisis.

Any new health care delivery system must go back to the basics. Those include good nutrition, regular exercise, and appropriate immunization. It should be a part of the curriculum of every school and the schedule of every adult.

In his terrific new book, *The Dakota Diet,* Dr. Weiland shares something that many Native Americans have known for centuries. A natural diet that emphasizes exercise, and the importance of lean meat like buffalo, fish, whole fruits and vegetables is the right thing to do, not only for one's health, but also for our environment.

Unfortunately, it may be many more years before our country adopts a new health care system. But a new health care discipline can begin right now. By adopting his recommendations for diet and a healthier lifestyle, every American can beat the national statistics and expect to live a longer and healthier life. That will affect not only your life, be the lives of others, too.

Follow Dr. Weiland's guidance in the pages of this book and you will feel better in more ways than one.

Tom Daschle
Former Representative and Senator from South Dakota (1979–2005),
and author of *Like No Other Time: The 107th Congress and the Two Years
That Changed America Forever* (Random House, 2003)

CHAPTER 1

The American State of Unhealth

As an internal medicine physician, I specialize in the health care of adults. Like a pediatrician with children, I focus on adults. I have made a career of treating health problems that certainly include diabetes and heart disease. But I am lucky to be practicing medicine in this modern age when we can foresee, detect, and prevent disease before it overcomes the patient.

Like many internists, preventive medicine is a major part of my practice. My journey to disease prevention actually began long before I started medical school. What I witnessed while growing up in a small town in South Dakota helped shape me into the physician I am today. My parents were hardworking owners and operators of a funeral home and ambulance service on the eastern side of the state. Back then, the local funeral homes typically provided the ambulance service since the hearse could easily transport the sick or injured to the hospital.

Not only did my father run the ambulance service, he was also one of the first emergency medical technicians (EMT) trained in the state. As an EMT, he had the necessary training in basic life support, but it was his experiences as a medic in World War II that gave him the confidence to care for the sick and injured. He was on call for our little community 24 hours a day, seven days a week, at a time when beepers and cell phones were pure science fiction. My mother served as his answering service and dispatcher. She alone had the responsibility of tracking down my father in the event someone needed his

1

help. Needless to say, the Weiland Ambulance Service was an integral part of the community.

Riding in the back of a hearse converted to an ambulance was quite an experience, especially for a 16-year-old boy. My job was to make the patient as comfortable as possible during the ride to the hospital. Just for the record, there is no comparing the smooth ride of a Cadillac hearse with today's ambulances built on the frames of one-ton trucks.

To this day, I vividly remember helping my father transport one patient out of a muddy corn field. It was late in the harvest season, and the farmer had been working frantically to get the last of his crops out before the first snow. When we arrived on the scene, he was sitting in an enclosed combine with his fist clenched tightly to his chest as he struggled to breathe. His skin was pale and clammy, and his eyes had a blank stare of death. He was in his mid-fifties and extremely overweight, and it took several of us to get him on a stretcher and into the back of the ambulance. In the emergency room, the doctor began to perform a new procedure for the time, known as CPR (cardiopulmonary resuscitation). After several laborious hours, the doctor pronounced the farmer dead. The autopsy determined the cause of death was a heart attack (myocardial infarction) and found that several arteries were blocked in his heart. The report also noted that the gentleman had diabetes and high blood pressure.

THE IMPORTANCE OF PREVENTIVE MEDICINE

The world has changed since those days, especially in field of medicine. Instead of teenagers, we now have paramedics with special training in the pre-hospital care of the sick and injured and ambulances are like rolling emergency rooms.

Not only has technology improved the standard of care for the sick and injured before they get to the hospital, it has also saved countless lives as a result of advances in the care of an acute coronary syndrome such as a heart attack. Hospitals today are staffed with individuals trained to administer life-saving medications upon a patient's arrival. Many hospitals have cardiologists on call, who can open up a coronary artery and spare a patient's heart from further damage.

The price tag for this type of care obviously has changed as well. While an ambulance trip in the 1970s cost $2, the same trip today could cost anywhere from $200 to $2,000. Emergency treatment for heart disease in the hospital can cost well over $20,000 for a single event—a tremendous expense for our society.

What remains unchanged are the risk factors that lead to heart disease in the first place. Just like the overweight farmer I cared for long ago, obesity in combination with a sedentary lifestyle has resulted in as many as 50 million Americans at risk for premature heart disease and death. The medical cost in treating diseases related to obesity has exceeded the cost of treating all of the diseases related to smoking.

To make an analogy, let's assume our government budgets $100 billion to clean up the Mississippi River. They decide that 90% of those dollars are to be spent cleaning the pollution out of the river down in New Orleans, when it would make more sense to focus those dollars on preventing the river from being polluted upstream. This is true for health care as well. Unfortunately, we spend nearly $2 trillion on health care in this country, with nearly 90% of this amount being spent to treat disease near the end of life. Very little is earmarked for prevention. The pollution that goes into the river (or the body) will manifest itself in disease unless we do more to educate ourselves and prevent this from happening.

I have dedicated my career to the prevention of disease and to educating my patients to practice a preventative approach, therefore saving them the expense and emotional toll of treating a disease. I have seen firsthand the diseases caused by our overindulgence in food as well as our sedentary culture. My hope is that in reading *The Dakota Diet*, you will gain a better understanding of what foods are important to eat and which ones to avoid. The goal is to prevent diseases associated with obesity, such as diabetes and high cholesterol. I see the effects of prevention working every day in my patient's lives as well as my own. I hope this book will have a positive impact on your health as well as your family's health.

THE PRICE OF EXCESS WEIGHT

Our current state of unhealth is costing us, in dollars and in ill health.

- The number of workdays lost due to illnesses attributable to excessive weight amounts to 53.6 million days per year. Employers lose an additional $4 billion annually in lost productivity. (*Shape Up America!*, March 1999)

- The health-care costs of treating seriously overweight adults in the U.S. in 1999 were estimated at $238 billion. (American Obesity Association, 1999)

- Over $100 billion is spent on medical expenses and loss of income due to weight conditions in the U.S. each year. This figure does not include the $47.6 billion spent per year to shed excess weight. (National Heart, Lung and Blood Institute, "Clinical Guidelines on Identification, Evaluation and Treatment of Overweight and Obesity in Adults," 1998)

- More than $51.6 billion is spent each year on health-care costs related to the cardiovascular complications of weight problems. (*Shape Up America!*, March 1999)

Health Implications

Excess weight is also a contributing factor in a number of serious illnesses.

- Being overweight is associated with heart disease, cancer, high blood pressure, high cholesterol, and diabetes, which are conditions that lead to disability and death in the United States. ("Guidance for Treatment of Adult Obesity," *Shape Up America!*, American Obesity Association, 1999, pp. 16–23)

- Conditions related to being seriously overweight contribute to 300,000 deaths every year, and are second only to smoking as a cause of preventable death. (*Journal of the American Medical Association* 1996; 276: 1907–1915)

- One-third of all cases of high blood pressure are associated with weight problems, and seriously overweight individuals are 50% more likely to have elevated blood cholesterol levels. (*American Family Physician* 1997; 55: 551–558)

- According to the American Diabetes Association, there are 16 million diabetics in the U.S. Of these, 15 million are type 2 diabetics, the form of diabetes that is closely associated with being overweight. ("Guidance for Treatment of Adult Obesity," *Shape Up America!*, American Obesity Association, 1999, p. 18)

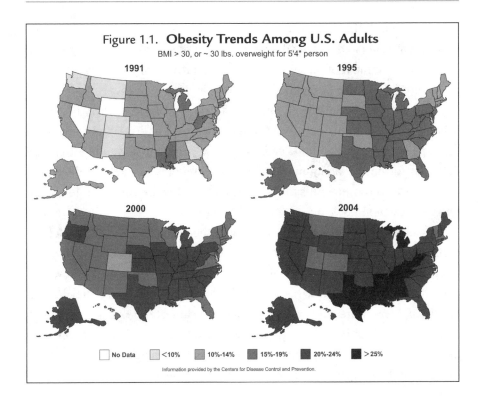

Figure 1.1. **Obesity Trends Among U.S. Adults**
BMI > 30, or ~ 30 lbs. overweight for 5'4" person

1991   1995

2000   2004

No Data   <10%   10%-14%   15%-19%   20%-24%   >25%

Information provided by the Centers for Disease Control and Prevention.

- Overweight men are more likely to die of colorectal or prostate cancers than non-overweight men, and overweight women are at greater risk of dying of endometrial, gallbladder, cervical, ovarian, and breast cancers than women without weight problems. (*American Family Physician* 1997; 55: 551–558)

- Gallstones occur three to six times more often in overweight people. Among women, 70% of gallstone cases are attributable to weight conditions. (*Shape Up America!*, December 1995)

THE CONFUSION OF POPULAR DIETS

Over the past several decades, the general public has been exposed to numerous diets in its attempt to lose weight. Even though some people achieve their desired weight loss, many regain the weight after stopping the diet. The major problem I have with these popular diets is the fact that they are based on eating plans that are not nutritionally sound. The Center for Science in the Public Interest, a consumer group that focuses on food and nutrition, recently met and reviewed several popular diet books. They came to the conclusion that most of these diet plans were nutritionally unacceptable.

One of the more popular diet trends has been the low-carbohydrate, high-protein, and high-fat diet. Dr. Robert Atkins's *Diet Revolution,* first published in 1972, and his *New Diet Revolution* (revised in 2001) both advocate this type of diet. His diet limits carbs so severely that the body starts to break down fat for energy and a metabolic condition known as ketosis develops. His diet is also too high in saturated fat and too low in fruits, whole grains, fiber, and calcium.

A diet high in saturated fats causes your body to produce too much low-density lipoprotein (LDL or "bad") cholesterol and reduces high-density lipoprotein (HDL or "good") cholesterol in the body. Recently, I followed a patient's attempt to lower his weight by following the Atkins diet. As his physician, I was more concerned with his high cholesterol than his weight as he had a fairly lean body base given his height. Interestingly enough, he lost his desired weight of 10 pounds. However, his LDL cholesterol went from a marginally dangerous level of 123 to an unsafe level of 210 after several months of dieting.

When the arteries in the body (including the arteries that supply nutrients to the heart muscle) are exposed to high levels of LDL cholesterol after a high-fat meal, they are predisposed to constricting as well as clotting. If blood flow is reduced or obstructed, a heart attack or stroke often occurs. LDL is actually a carrier protein in the blood that delivers cholesterol to the cells in the body for use in the cell wall or to make hormones. If you have high levels of LDL, the carrier protein will dump its unused cargo (cholesterol) onto the walls of the artery, resulting in plaque formation (arteriosclerosis).

Another patient I recently cared for was told by his physician that he was "pre-diabetic" because of obesity. He was so upset by the news that he took it upon himself to lose weight. He followed the Atkins diet and lost 10 pounds in the first month. I met him when he was admitted to the hospital and to my medical service with a condition known as acute pancreatitis. That morning, he had his usual large portion of bacon and eggs, but then developed abdominal pain. His pain was so severe that he had to be admitted to the hospital. His blood triglycerides (fats formed from the fats in food) were 10 times their normal level, causing his pancreas to react violently, becoming inflamed. The pancreas is the organ where insulin is produced. When inflamed (pancreatitis), pancreatic cells are destroyed and no longer able to produce insulin—as was the case in this unfortunate patient.

Another consequence of eating a high-fat, high-protein diet is that fiber is also severely restricted. Constipation can result if this very important food group is eliminated in the diet. Constipation can even flare up a diverticulum in the colon, causing a potential serious medical condition known as diverticulitis. Diverticuli are sacs or pouches within the colon that are formed when the walls of the large bowel are weakened.

The book *Protein Power* by Drs. Michael R. Eades and Mary Dan Eades, published in 1996, focuses on a high-protein, low-carbohydrate diet as a way to lose weight. Again, the problem is in the amount of saturated fat consumed and that the diet is high in protein. Another patient of mine chose to eat a high-protein diet and, as a result, he developed acute gouty arthritis. Gout is an inflammatory condition of the joints in which a chemical called uric acid causes small crystals to form in the joint. These crystals are responsible for the inflammation and pain associated with acute gouty arthritis. The uric acid that accumulates in the blood and joints is a result of breaking down certain proteins consumed in the diet. The kidneys may also be affected, resulting in kidney stones made of uric acid.

Most of the popular diets seem to focus on carbohydrates as solely responsible for weight gain and many of these diets feature high-fat foods. Granted, fat has been shown to cause early satiety (feelings of fullness), resulting in less food consumed, but the health consequences from such a diet may be irreversible.

Just as Atkins was the grandfather of low-carb dieting, Dr. Robert Pritikin is considered by most nutritionists as the grandfather of low-fat dieting. His book *The Pritikin Principle,* published in 2000, features a diet that includes limited amounts of poultry, seafood, and meats, but generous servings of carbohydrates in the form of vegetables, pastas, and fruits. Those who have tried it that I have spoken to found it very difficult to limit their fat intake. What Pritikin did not know was that not all fats are bad fats. We know today that certain fats, such as omega-3 fatty acids (found in many foods, including canola oil, range-fed buffalo, and salmon), can actually improve your cholesterol profile by raising the HDL and lowering LDL.

More recently, Dr. Dean Ornish's 2001 book *Eat More, Weigh Less* is a diet that severely restricts fat and allows a liberal consumption of carbohydrates. While in my internal medicine residency at the University of Wisconsin in Madison, I attempted to restrict the fat in my diet. I increased my fiber and carbohydrate intake, but never really lost weight and felt hungry most of the time. It was not until later in my professional career that I learned that fat leaves the stomach very slowly, reducing food cravings. Thus, a certain amount of fat may actually help you lose weight.

The Zone (1995) by Barry Sears attempts to control insulin levels through a diet low in fat but with plenty of fresh fruits and vegetables. I had the pleasant opportunity of meeting Dr. Sears at a medical conference recently and he piqued my interest in the importance of healthy dieting. He recommends a meal plan that is very simple to follow. All you have to do is fill your plate with one-third protein and two-thirds fruits and vegetables.

I was equally impressed with Dr. Arthur Agatstons' book *The South Beach Diet* (2003). I found his approach to dieting easy to follow, and like Dr. Sears, he advocates the right amount of fats, protein, and carbohydrates. His chapter on how to eat in a restaurant provides a few tricks to help you choose the right foods on the menu as well as other tips to assure that you eat less.

Both Drs. Agatston and Sears advocate complex carbohydrates as well as a balance of fats and protein. Consuming these types of foods is how we are designed genetically to sustain our bodies. By eating more refined foods, such as white rice and baked goods, the body processes the carbohydrate easily—raising the blood sugar too quickly. The pancreas then responds by secreting high levels of insulin, driving the blood sugar down too rapidly. This will tend to leave you craving another carbohydrate within an hour or two of eating a simple carbohydrate.

In my quest for the perfect diet, my wife (also a physician) introduced me to Dr. Artemis Simopoulos' book *The Omega Diet* (1999). Based on a nutritional program from the Island of Crete, her book focuses on the health benefits of omega-3 fatty acids. She does a wonderful job explaining the benefits of consuming foods rich in omega-3s and her book is worth reading for anyone interested in the real science behind omega-3 fatty acids.

As I was reading Dr. Simopoulos's book, the first thing that came to mind was buffalo. The meat of the buffalo that graze on the plains of the Dakotas has a lower amount of saturated fat and cholesterol and a higher level of omega-3 fats than their feedlot counterparts. I was so inspired by what I was reading that I decided to develop a diet plan for my own patients who are battling the American belly bulge and high cholesterol. My first test subject was none other then myself. By watching what I was eating and increasing my activity, I not only lost weight, I lowered my total cholesterol by 25 points, lowered my bad cholesterol from 135 to 106, and raised my good cholesterol from 45 to 61. I switched from eating beef high in saturated fat to leaner, grass-fed buffalo.

The term *dieting* should not be associated with losing weight. Weight loss is only one benefit—lowering your blood pressure and blood cholesterol are other, more important consequences. Fad dieting is just that—a fad that comes and goes as fast as your weight does. A healthy diet is not a fad diet but rather a diet with the right amounts and types of food in order to achieve and maintain a desired weight. When combined with physical activity, the health benefits will continue for years.

HOW TO KICK YOUR METABOLISM INTO HIGH GEAR

Most people have good intentions when starting a weight loss program, but often end up abandoning their New Year's resolution of shedding a few pounds. In fact, only one out of 100 dieters will lose the weight they want to permanently. Many diets fail because it is nearly impossible to continue to eat the same foods every day. Another reason for failure is the lack of physical activity, which can lower your metabolism.

Metabolism is the sum of all the chemical and physical changes in the body that enable its continued growth and function. Simply put, it is a means by which the body uses energy (calories) in order to function properly. The body needs a minimum amount of energy to maintain vital functions, such as breathing, digestion, and blood circulation. This is referred to as your basal metabolic rate (BMR). As we age, our metabolism slows by about 2% per year and most of us gain a few pounds and find weight loss harder to achieve.

Weight loss medications claim to boost your metabolism in order to achieve weight loss—with very little effort on your part. Many of these so-called miracle pills contain a drug called ephedrine, which acts like adrenaline in the body, speeding up metabolism. (Ephedra, also called ma huang, is a naturally occurring substance derived from plants; ephedrine is a synthetic derivative.) The drug was banned for a time by the U.S. Food and Drug Administration when it was reported that it was linked to heart attacks and strokes. The good news is that you can improve your metabolism safely by simply eating right and exercising.

Yes, food can increase your metabolism. Many diets fail because they restrict calories to the point where your metabolism slows, making it more difficult to lose weight. When the body is starving for calories (energy), it conserves fat and slows metabolism in an attempt to survive. Eventually, the body begins to break down (catabolism) vital tissue, such as muscle protein, for fuel. The immediate weight loss noticed is the loss of water weight as the body attempts to flush away a by-product of protein catabolism—nitrogen—through the kidneys. The water weight quickly returns as soon as you replenish the fluids, but the muscle wasting will continue as long as you restrict your calories.

Once you start to lose muscle mass, your BMR changes as well. One pound of muscle will burn 50 calories a day at rest. Dieters can lose up to 1 pound of muscle for every 3 pounds of fat by restricting the fuel the body needs in order to function. If a dieter loses 5 pounds of muscle, he or she must consume 250 fewer calories a day in order to maintain their weight loss. Additionally, thyroid hormone production may decrease, resulting in an even slower metabolism. When the dieter returns to their old ways, the weight quickly returns in the form of fat, with less muscle mass than they had before they started the diet.

The real key to a successful weight loss is kicking your metabolism into high gear through aerobic exercise, strength training, and eating the right foods. Strength training with either free weights or resistance bands (at least twice a week) can boost your metabolism and keep it high for many hours after a workout. Aerobic activity such as walking, jogging, cycling, or swimming for 30 minutes a day, three to four times a week, is also essential for successful weight loss. And don't forget to eat—research suggests that eating small meals frequently can boost metabolism and help you lose weight.

The goal for any diet is to maintain lean body mass while losing body fat.

It is possible to gain 1 pound of muscle for every pound of fat lost. Obviously, the scale will not change, but the pant or dress size will. Remember, a healthy diet is not a fad diet; rather, it is a diet with the right amounts and types of food in order to achieve and maintain a desired weight. When combined with physical activity, the health benefits will continue for years.

A SIMPLE SOLUTION

Millions of people in this country have been struggling to lose weight. It seems all too often that society wants the "slim fast" program for weight loss. That's why the fad diet plans continue to be popular and these books continue to appear at the top of the best-seller lists. In addition to these diet plans, pharmaceutical companies have also gotten involved in the quest for weight loss, marketing medications to help control appetite and other drugs that actually block the amount of fat absorbed. Natural product industries have made billions of dollars on rapid weight loss products containing a synthetic ephedra-like substance to increase your metabolism and suppress appetite.

Despite billions of dollars spent for weight loss, we have become one of the fattest nations in the world. Because of obesity, we have spent even more money on diet-related diseases, such as diabetes, high blood pressure, and sleep apnea. Physicians understand how important weight is when dealing with the health of their patients. The reality is that most patients will have a difficult time losing weight and keeping the weight off without a major lifestyle change. The "slim fast" program for weight loss is only a temporary fix and life would be very boring if you had to follow a fad diet plan for the rest of your life.

My solution for weight loss is a simple one: reduce your daily calorie intake and increase your metabolism by exercise. You will not only lose the necessary weight for ideal health, you will also improve your cardiovascular profile by lowering your cholesterol and blood pressure. Studies sponsored by the U.S. Centers for Disease Control and Prevention (CDC) and the National Institutes of Health (NIH) have shown that this works. Despite the overwhelming research on obesity, our food industry still dictates what types of food we eat. The CDC and NIH as well as the American Heart Association have made their recommendations to our congressional leaders, asking their support to fund programs designed to prevent obesity. The Improved Nutrition and Physical Activity (IMPACT) Act, which was introduced in the Senate several years ago, addresses obesity prevention in schools by promoting physical activity and good nutrition in young people. We have seen obesity rates in young people double in the last 20 years and, as a result, we have witnessed increases in type 2 diabetes, high cholesterol, and high blood pressure.

I lost my weight the "slim slow" way. By reducing my calories and increasing my activity, I was able to achieve a healthy weight as well as improve my cholesterol profile. I coined the term *Dakota Diet* because my plan features buffalo as well as other foods produced right in the heart of the Dakotas. Based on the concept of the Mediterranean Diet, the Dakota Diet is high in good fats (especially omega-3 fatty acids) found in abundance in flax seed, soy, buffalo, and wild game. It is also high in soluble fiber found in beans, barley and oats, which also contain beta-glucans, substances that interfere with the absorption of cholesterol in your diet.

The following chapters provide all the details of my diet plan. The next chapter looks at the basics of nutrition, with a special emphasis on exploring the difference between good fats and bad fats, which is the emphasis of my plan. Chapter 3: Healthy Foods From the Dakotas looks at the variety of healthy foods available right here in the Great Plains, including grass-fed buffalo, of course—all part of the Dakota Diet. Chapter 4 gets into the nitty-gritty details of my diet, including shopping and cooking tips as well as a 14-day meal plan. Chapter 5: Get Fit and Stay Slim looks at the importance of exercise and physical activity to weight loss. And Chapter 6: The Dakota Diet and Disease Prevention examines the links between the healthy foods in the Dakota Diet and preventing diseases such as high cholesterol, heart disease, and diabetes.

The Dakota Diet is not a fad diet—rather, it is a way of eating that provides you with the proper nutrients in order to live healthier.

CHAPTER 2

The Basics
of Good Nutrition

One can only imagine what the Great Plains of the Dakotas might have looked like hundreds of years ago—a land rich in buffalo and abundant with wild grasses. In order to survive, you would have had to gather and hunt your food, consuming only what was necessary. For the indigenous people roaming the land, this was their way of life for over a thousand years.

The human body is genetically programmed to adjust to the environment and develop the most efficient means of subsistence. During times of feasting, the body stored the extra calories consumed by making them into fat. When food was not as plentiful, the body would then tap into those reserves, thus providing the necessary calories to endure. It took thousands of years to develop such an efficient way to survive on this earth. As a result, even today we are programmed to thrive on a diet similar to those of the Plains Indians.

Unfortunately, what is happening in America today is that every meal is a feast and the only time we fast is when we sleep. We interrupt our fasting between meals with a high-carbohydrate snack and "hunt" for our food by pushing a large metal cage with wheels around the grocery aisles. We do very little "gathering" in the form of exercise and consume enough calories in one meal to run a 5K race. However, our genetic makeup has not changed, so, as a result, we are efficiently storing the excessive calories consumed when we super-size our fries.

The Plains Indians had a healthy lifestyle, but then the buffalo were gone and they were confined to reservations. No longer able to hunt, and for their survival, they were given commodities such as refined flour—thus, the creation of "Indian fry bread." One serving of this flat bread (1 to 3 ounces) provided them with 325 calories and a large dose of simple carbohydrates. Hunting and gathering became a thing of the past and their new diet resulted in obesity, diabetes, heart disease, and premature death. Sound familiar?

Can we change the unhealthy path we are on? Well, the answer might be right here in America's back yard.

GETTING BACK TO THE ORIGINAL DIET

The original diet of the Plains Indians was one of foods rich in omega-3 fatty acids and less of the omega-6 fatty acids. These fatty acids are considered essential fats our body needs and can only be obtained in the diet. Both types play key roles in our health by converting a substance called eicosanoids into hormones that influence or suppress our immune system and affect our perception of pain and inflammation. Today, our diet contains very low levels of omega-3s. As we forage for food at the grocery store, the food that we bring home contains up to 20 times more omega-6s than omega-3s. A healthy ratio of omega-6 to omega-3 should be around 4 to 1.

Grazing animals that are allowed to eat a natural diet of plants are far richer in omega-3 fatty acids than a confined animal fed a grain-based diet. The Plains Indians ate large quantities of animal protein, mostly buffalo meat, but it contained healthier fats than the meats we generally consume today. Not only did the Indians eat a diet rich in animal protein, they also consumed up to four times more fruits and vegetables then we do today. Cereals and grains were a source of energy for the Plains Indians; however, these two food groups where naturally rich in fiber and other complex carbohydrates, as opposed to the simple carbohydrates so common in the modern diet.

As we have modernized our own diet and lifestyle, our consumption of omega-3 fatty acids has been significantly reduced and has been replaced by omega-6 fats. Omega-6s are found in vegetable oils such as corn, safflower, sunflower, and cottonseed. They are the precursors of arachidonic acid, a fatty acid that is part of the inflammatory cascade in the body. Research has shown that silent inflammation can be a predictor for heart disease, strokes, and premature aging in the cells of the body. Therefore, you may put yourself at risk for disease by consuming a diet high in omega-6 fatty acids and subsequently increasing these inflammatory acids in the body.

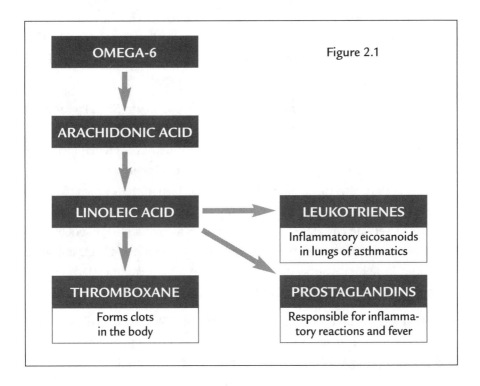

Omega-3s counter the omega-6 fatty acids and are found abundantly in foods from the plains of the Dakotas. The Dakota Diet features buffalo and other range-fed animals such as chicken and wild game. It is low in simple carbohydrates and high in omega-3 fatty acids as well as complex carbohydrates such as soluble fiber (found in beans, oats, and barley). It is a diet that is nutritionally sound and, when combined with the proper exercise, not only will help you lose weight, it will improve your cholesterol profile and add more, healthier years to your life.

BALANCING THE MACRONUTRIENTS

"You are what you eat" as the old saying goes. Diets that severely limit or recommend in excess any of these basic macronutrients—carbohydrates, fats, and protein—can put your health at risk. For example, a diet high in protein can cause harm to the kidneys and has been linked to cancers of the colon. Too much fat in the diet leads to heart disease as well as a multitude of other cancers. Too many carbohydrates can lead to diabetes and obesity.

A commonsense guideline for any weight loss (or weight control) program is to balance these macronutrients. If weight loss is your goal, then reduce your total intake of calories for the day and increase your expenditure of calories through exercise.

- Your total carbohydrate intake should range from 45% to 55% of your daily calories. Again, I remind you that fiber is a carbohydrate and avoiding healthy carbs such as fiber can cause a multitude of problems, including constipation. Carbohydrates are a great source of energy and are important for a well-balanced diet. The old U.S. Department of Agriculture (USDA) food pyramid was confusing in that it recommended that you eat six to 11 servings of grains or grain products a day. One bagel equates to roughly five servings of grain (as well as 350 calories). If you are on a 2,000-calorie diet, you would meet or exceed the recommended requirement of carbohydrate after your third bagel.

- Protein intake should range between 20% and 25% of your daily calories. Protein comes from meat, eggs, dairy, and nuts. I recommend protein with every meal, as it will help reduce your hunger between meals.

Calories in Macronutrients

One gram of carbohydrate = 4 calories · One gram of protein = 4 calories · One gram of fat = 9 calories

- The exciting news to most people is our greater understanding of good fats and bad fats, which is the basis of this book. Your diet should consist of a total fat intake around 25% to 35% of daily calories, with less than 7% coming from saturated fat. The grass-fed animals of the Dakotas are not only a great source of nutrient-dense, low-calorie protein, they are also low in saturated fat and higher in healthy omega-3 fatty acids.

THE FACTS ON FATS

The next time you shop for food at your local grocery store, spend some time reading the nutritional labels of the products you buy. (See Figure 2.2 below.) Pay attention not only to the amount of carbohydrates and calories per serving, but also focus on the amount and types of fats the food contains as well. You will be surprised to learn what you are eating in the form of fats.

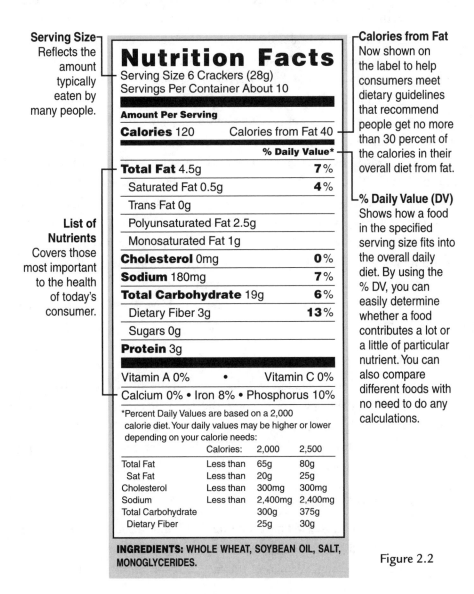

Serving Size Reflects the amount typically eaten by many people.

Nutrition Facts

Serving Size 6 Crackers (28g)
Servings Per Container About 10

Amount Per Serving

Calories 120   Calories from Fat 40

% Daily Value*

Total Fat 4.5g	**7**%
Saturated Fat 0.5g	**4**%
Trans Fat 0g	
Polyunsaturated Fat 2.5g	
Monosaturated Fat 1g	
Cholesterol 0mg	**0**%
Sodium 180mg	**7**%
Total Carbohydrate 19g	**6**%
Dietary Fiber 3g	**13**%
Sugars 0g	
Protein 3g	

Vitamin A 0%   •   Vitamin C 0%

Calcium 0% • Iron 8% • Phosphorus 10%

*Percent Daily Values are based on a 2,000 calorie diet. Your daily values may be higher or lower depending on your calorie needs:

	Calories:	2,000	2,500
Total Fat	Less than	65g	80g
Sat Fat	Less than	20g	25g
Cholesterol	Less than	300mg	300mg
Sodium	Less than	2,400mg	2,400mg
Total Carbohydrate		300g	375g
Dietary Fiber		25g	30g

INGREDIENTS: WHOLE WHEAT, SOYBEAN OIL, SALT, MONOGLYCERIDES.

Calories from Fat Now shown on the label to help consumers meet dietary guidelines that recommend people get no more than 30 percent of the calories in their overall diet from fat.

% Daily Value (DV) Shows how a food in the specified serving size fits into the overall daily diet. By using the % DV, you can easily determine whether a food contributes a lot or a little of particular nutrient. You can also compare different foods with no need to do any calculations.

List of Nutrients Covers those most important to the health of today's consumer.

Figure 2.2

Before the low-carbohydrate diet fad, most nutritionists believed that the way to lose weight was to avoid fats. By simply stripping away the fats from your diet, you would lose weight by boosting your metabolism. Subsequently, the food industry followed suit and started to produce numerous low-fat and fat-free products.

Most of us were duped into thinking that "fat free" meant calorie free and we could eat an unlimited amount without gaining weight. As we started to reduce the amount of fat in our diets, our carbohydrate consumption increased as did our total calories. Instead of losing the necessary weight by burning fat, we became fat machines by converting the excess carbohydrates into fat. To make matters worse, the type of fat produced is a saturated fat that has been linked to high cholesterol and heart disease.

Fatty acids are components of fats and oils. They differ from each other by the placement of molecular bonds and the number of carbon atoms they contain. Research into diet and weight loss has surprisingly shown that it is not dietary fat that makes you fat—rather, it is the amount of calories and lack of exercise that makes you fat. Further research has shown that not all fats are bad for you and the types of fats we consume in our diet can have a profound effect on our health. In simpler terms, our body needs a certain amount of fat for optimal health. The Dakota Diet provides you with the right type by featuring foods that are rich in omega-3 fats.

Here are the common types of fats or fatty acids we consume through the diet (see Table 2.1):

Saturated Fats

Saturated fatty acids are loaded with hydrogen atoms to the point that they cannot accommodate any more—thus, the term *saturated*. Most of these types of fats or oils are solid at room temperature. Animal fat and butter fat are examples of saturated fats. Saturated fats have been shown to raise blood cholesterol, putting you at risk for heart disease and strokes.

Monounsaturated Fats

Monounsaturated fatty acids have one double bond in the fatty acid chain and are liquid at room temperature. Examples of monounsaturated oils are canola oil and olive oil (over 85% of the fatty acids in these popular oils are monounsaturated). These types of fats can improve your cholesterol profile by raising your good (high-density lipoprotein or HDL) cholesterol and lowering your bad (low-density lipoprotein or LDL) cholesterol. For this reason, I recommend these types of oils as your main cooking oils.

Polyunsaturated Fats

Polyunsaturated fatty acids have two or more double bonds in their chain. They are liquid at room temperature and remain in their liquid form in the refrigerator. (The more double bonds on the carbon chain, the more unsaturated the oil and the less likely the oil will thicken when refrigerated.) Flaxseed oil and fish oils are the most highly unsaturated of all oils. These types of fatty acids are heart healthy because they can lower your LDL (bad) cholesterol and raise your HDL (good) cholesterol.

Trans-Fatty Acids

Trans-fatty acids (TFAs) are partially hydrogenated vegetable oils, such as corn oil, found in margarines and other convenience foods. Processed foods contain this type of oil because it increases product shelf-life. As a result of hydrogenation (adding a hydrogen molecule to the chain of carbons), trans-fatty acids behave in many ways like saturated fats and can actually be even more destructive by raising your LDL and lowering your HDL. French fries, doughnuts, cookies, chips, and other snack food are high in trans-fatty acids. In fact, nearly all fried or baked goods have some form of trans-fatty acids. So, switching from butter to margarine is not such a good idea after all.

TABLE 2.1. FATTY ACIDS AND THEIR EFFECTS		
Type of Fatty Acid	**Examples**	**Effects on the Body**
Saturated fat	Animal fat	Raises LDL (bad) cholesterol, lowers HDL (good) cholesterol
Monounsaturated fat	Olive oil, canola oil	Lowers LDL (bad) cholesterol, raises HDL (good) cholesterol
Polyunsaturated fat	Flax seed, fish oil	Lowers LDL (bad) cholesterol, raises HDL (good) cholesterol
Trans-fatty acid	Margarine	Raises LDL (bad) cholesterol, lowers HDL (good) cholesterol

THE IMPORTANCE OF ESSENTIAL FATTY ACIDS

Omega-3 and omega-6 oils are polyunsaturated oils. Omega-3 fatty acids have their first double bond between the third and fourth carbon atoms and are called omega-3s. Omega-6 fatty acids have their first double bond between the sixth and seventh carbon atoms, hence the designation "omega-6." Oils such as corn, safflower, sunflower, and peanut are high in omega-6s, whereas oils such as canola, walnut, and flaxseed are high in omega-3s. Omega-3 fatty acids and omega-6 fatty acids are considered "essential" fatty acids in that they cannot be manufactured within the body—they can only be obtained from the diet.

Our body eventually converts these important acids into other types of acids called eicosanoids. The eicosanoids produced by omega-3 and omega-6 fatty acids have opposite functions in the body. New research into the polyunsaturated oils has shown that the ratio of omega-6 to omega-3 fats in your diet can have dramatically different effects on your health.

First, one has to understand how these fats are converted to the hormone-like substances that actually influence functions in your body. The primary fatty acid in the omega 6 family is called linoleic acid and the primary omega-3 fat is alpha-linolenic acid. When these essential fatty acids are consumed, they interact with certain enzymes in the body. As a result of this chemical reaction, they become desaturated by losing a hydrogen atom, which increases the number of double bonds in their chain. The chain also becomes longer by adding more carbon atoms.

If your diet is high in omega-6 oils, your body will produce more of the type of eicosanoids that can increase your risk for inflammation and the development of asthma and allergies—linoleic acid converts to arachidonic acid, which in turn is converted to leukotrienes. Leukotrienes are inflammatory substances found in the lungs of those with asthma. When an asthma attack occurs, these eicosanoids can increase up to three times higher than normal in the lungs of asthmatics. Steroids, commonly used to treat asthmatic patients, block the production of leukotrienes. As mentioned before, omega-3 fatty acids work in opposition to omega-6s, also blocking the production of these inflammatory hormones in the lung.

In addition to higher levels of leukotrienes, two other eicosanoids are formed as a result of too much omega-6 in your diet: prostaglandins, which can lead to increased inflammation, and thromboxanes, which can increase the risk for blood clots. Clotting, for obvious reasons, is important to help stop bleeding when you cut yourself, but it is when we form clots within the blood vessels that disease of the heart and brain occurs. People at high risk for these problems are given an aspirin a day in order to block the formation of thromboxane. Therefore, a diet high in omega-3 fatty acids will also help slow abnormal blood clotting in the body.

Prostaglandins are hormones that play a crucial role in the body's response to inflammation. They are produced and released by nearly every cell in the body, with the exception of red blood cells. When arachidonic acid interacts with the enzyme cyclo-oxygenase, prostaglandins are formed. The hormone-like affect of prostaglandins results in inflammatory reactions, causing pain and fevers. For example, when a woman experiences menstrual pain (dysmenorrhea), prostaglandins are overproduced during menstruation causing a lot of discomfort. Aspirin and other anti-inflammatory drugs, such as ibuprofen or naproxen, short-circuit the production of prostaglandins and relieve the menstrual pain. A diet high in omega-3 fatty acids (as in the Dakota Diet) will have a similar effect, resulting in less discomfort during menstruation.

The body needs a balance of the essential fatty acids. An inflammatory response is an important part of fighting infections and it is equally critical to stop the bleeding when we cut ourselves, so we need the eicosanoids. It is when the diet is overloaded with omega-6s and deficient in omega-3s that disease occurs. The typical American diet has a ratio of omega-6 to omega-3 of 20 to 1. A healthy balance should be around 4 to 1.

Deficiencies of omega-3 fatty acids have also been linked to impulsive and aggressive behavior in adults as well as children. Another consequence of growing up deficient in omega-3s is attention-deficit/hyperactivity disorder (ADHD). Studies have shown that boys with ADHD have significantly lower levels of two hormone by-products of omega-3 fatty acids. Yet another study found that rats fed a diet deficient in omega-3s had less synaptic vesicles (pouches in the brain that store neurotransmitter chemicals needed for neurons to communicate). Their counterparts fed a diet enriched with omega-3 resulted in more synaptic vesicles and improved learning.

THE TRUTH ABOUT TRANS-FAT

Have you ever wondered why processed food items such as potato chips or crackers have an uncanny ability to sit on the grocery shelf for months on end without spoiling? It is not the wonderful packaging that keeps the chips so fresh—rather, it is the type of fat used in making the product that allows it to be preserved for extended periods of time.

The fat used in food preservation is actually a synthetic product developed from research by the French in the 1800s. In order to feed the hungry masses, Napoleon III encouraged French scientists to develop ways to help with food storage and spoilage problems. During this time, Louis Pasteur devised techniques in sterilization that not only revolutionized the field of surgery but also the wine industry, a process that came to be known as "pasteurization." Pasteurization is still used today to safeguard many foods and beverages, including milk.

What eventually emerged from this research forever changed the way food is preserved. By the end of the 19th century, a process called hydrogenation (which added a hydrogen molecule) was patented. Scientists were able to partially hydrogenate vegetable oil, which made it solid at room temperature. This "margarine" was sweeter and cleaner than other oils made from animal fat. By the 1950s, the hydrogenation of oils to make margarine made it the most popular table spread used in the United States.

It seemed a strange coincidence that the American Heart Association announced an increase in heart disease among adults in the United States at approximately the same time. The cause for this sudden increase was a mystery at the time. Today, heart disease is the number one killer in America and research into the consumption of this synthetic hydrogenated fat, known as trans-fatty acids, suggests a strong link to heart disease and strokes.

Over the past 20 years, independent researchers from Harvard and throughout the world have documented the potential dangers of TFAs in our diet. The Institute of Medicine at the National Academy of Sciences has advised the U.S. Food and Drug Administration (FDA) to alert the public to the presence of this harmful ingredient in our processed foods. The FDA now requires product labeling on all manufactured foods containing TFAs as of 2006. They also noted that nearly 40% of all supermarket foods contain TFAs, as do most fast foods and bakery goods.

The fact that TFAs are a major source of fat in our diet is not the only reason we have an epidemic of heart disease and diabetes in America today. Contributing factors include smoking, sedentary lifestyles, and genetics. TFAs, however, contribute to heart disease by increasing low-density lipoproteins in the blood. LDLs are the carrier proteins of cholesterol to the cells of the body and are responsible for the buildup of plaque in arteries. Trans-fatty acids increase LDL (bad) cholesterol and lower HDL (good) cholesterol. The first step in lowering your blood LDLs is to avoid all TFAs in your diet. Eliminating processed foods containing TFAs can help you control your cholesterol profile, especially if you have high LDL levels.

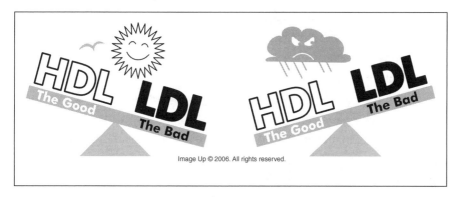

Figure 2.3

It will be difficult to determine which foods contain TFAs until the food industry labels all processed foods with the types and amounts of TFAs they contain. Even now, the FDA allows a company to claim their food is "trans-fat free" even if it contains up to 0.5 grams of partially hydrogenated soybeans. This is misleading and my advice is not only to read the label but also to look for TFAs in the product ingredients list before purchasing the item.

> Trans-fatty acids increase LDL (bad) cholesterol and lower HDL (good) cholesterol.

THERE IS NOTHING SIMPLE ABOUT CARBOHYDRATES

For me, growing up in a large family was essentially survival of the fittest— eat or be eaten, so to speak. Fortunately, our mother allowed us in the kitchen to prepare some of our own meals. I remember when my brother and I helped make our favorite treat, Nestlé Toll House chocolate chip cookies. The project soon took a turn for the worse as we ate half of the mixed ingredients while waiting for the oven to warm up. We were so full of raw cookie dough that we couldn't enjoy the taste of a hot, moist cookie dipped into a glass of ice cold milk. We finished the job eventually and enjoyed the fruits of our labor at a later date.

Our mother not only taught us how to follow a recipe and measure ingredients, she even allowed us to be creative enough to invent a few of our own recipes, most of which only the family dog could (and would) enjoy. One of our obnoxious concoctions consisted of a mixture of white flour and warm water. What impressed me about mixing these two ingredients was how easily the refined white flour dissolved in the water, producing a milky-looking fluid. We convinced our youngest brother that this is how milk was made and he should give it a try.

We then took equal amounts of stone-ground whole-wheat flour in an attempt to make a chocolate milk substitute. However, this combination did not mix very well. In fact, most of the ingredients either floated to the top or sank to the bottom of the glass. As a child, what I learned from these experiments is that my dog would eat just about anything we made and my little brother would believe just about everything we said. On the other hand, as a physician, my childhood experiments in the kitchen gave me a better understanding of simple and complex carbohydrates.

First of all, remember that all carbohydrates are made up of sugars. When consumed, our body begins to break down the carbohydrate into simple sugars. This is true for all carbohydrates, whether it is a refined grain (such as white rice or white bread) or a complex carbohydrate (such as a whole-grain health food cracker). Either way, the end product will always be the same—glucose. Glucose is your body's fuel, and cells use it to produce energy to grow and function properly.

Avoid simple carbohydrates such as white flour, sugars, and pastries. When wheat is refined and made into flour, the fiber is stripped away, making the carbohydrate or sugars in the flour much more easily absorbed in the digestive system (like my example of white flour dissolving in warm water). As a result, foods that are made of white flour, such as white bread, are simple carbohydrates that cause our blood sugar to spike rapidly. When we eat a whole-grain product, a complex carbohydrate with the fiber preserved, this slows down the amount of carbohydrate or sugar absorbed, resulting in a lower blood sugar rise in the body.

Once the sugars enter the bloodstream, the pancreas kicks in by producing the appropriate amount of insulin. Insulin is a hormone that allows glucose to enter the cell for use as energy, thus lowering your blood sugar. What the body does not use for energy will either be stored as unused glucose in the form of fat or be eliminated.

The bottom line is that a sharp rise in blood sugar results in a sharp rise in insulin, which will quickly drive the blood sugar levels down. If the blood sugar is driven down too far (reactive hypoglycemia), then the body responds by an overwhelming craving of more carbs in order to correct the problem. Eating more will result in more calories consumed and more weight gain. The pancreas also produces a hormone called glucagon in response to low blood sugar levels. This hormone taps into glucose stores in the liver in order to bring the blood sugar back to normal.

Choose healthy carbohydrates such as multigrain breads, whole fruits, and vegetables. By eating carbohydrates that are slowly absorbed (complex carbohydrates), insulin is slowly released and the drop in blood sugar is less drastic. If you have better control of your blood sugar, then you will have fewer cravings for carbohydrates, which results in fewer calories consumed.

But can you have your cake and eat it too? You bet, but only if you do this infrequently, never right before you go to bed, and only if you exercise. I have my own family now and, on a rare occasion, I will go back to mom's chocolate chip cookie recipe and bake a batch with my daughter. Like my mother, my wife and I have allowed her to create some of her own recipes. I can only predict what is in store for her two younger siblings and the family dog once we allow her full rein of the kitchen.

FIBER, "NATURES Q-TIP"

Here is a subject that remains off limits to most people—constipation. Comedians often find this topic a good source for a joke or two. If you order prunes or bran cereal for breakfast, you are sure to get a few comments and even some smirks. Unfortunately, over 4 million Americans suffer from constipation and it can be an embarrassing struggle, interfering with the quality of your life.

Constipation is a symptom, not a disease: like a fever, constipation can be caused by many different conditions. These may include a problem with the bowel itself, such as irritable bowel syndrome, hemorrhoids, or even cancer. Other health problems, such as an underactive thyroid and long-standing diabetes, can slow things down, causing constipation. There are many drugs with side effects of constipation, including narcotic derivatives (codeine and morphine used for pain control), high blood pressure medications (especially calcium channel blockers such as Adalat and Calan), diuretics (water pills), and antihistamines.

The most common cause of constipation is a diet low in the kinds of fiber found in vegetables, fruits, and whole grains, and high in fats found in processed foods, cheeses, and meats. As people attempt to lose weight by avoiding carbohydrates as is recommended with the Atkins diet, constipation can become a serious problem.

Fiber is a carbohydrate with a low glycemic index (GI); that is, it doesn't cause a dramatic blood sugar spike. Avoiding fiber in order to reduce your carbohydrates will put you at risk of developing constipation. The Dakota Diet is built around foods with a low glycemic index and high in fiber, therefore your chance of developing constipation is less. Fiber (both soluble and insoluble) is the part of fruits, vegetables, and grains that the body cannot digest. Soluble fiber dissolves easily in water and takes on a soft, gel-like texture in the intestines. Insoluble fiber passes almost unchanged through the intestines. The bulk and soft texture of fiber help prevent hard, dry stools that are difficult to pass.

TABLE 2.2. RECOMMENDED DAILY FIBER INTAKE		
Sex	**Age**	**Fiber**
Female	Under 50	25 g
Male	Under 50	38 g
Female	50 & over	21 g
Male	50 & over	30 g

Add a fiber supplement such as a bulk-forming agent in the form of psyllium (Metamucil, Fibercon) or a cellulose derivative such a Citrucel. They are safe over the long term, but may lead to increased bloating and gas until your body gets used to them. Avoid the use of harsh laxatives on a regular basis without your doctor's approval. Some of them might actually damage your colon and worsen the condition. Stool softeners like docusate (Colace and Surfak) and bulk agents are safer.

When you are adding extra fiber to your diet, drink at least eight ounces of water six times a day. Be aware that drinking water alone is not enough to prevent constipation and, without fiber, the water is absorbed quickly and the excess is excreted as urine.

If your constipation does not respond to simple measures or your symptoms persist longer than six weeks, you should see your doctor to sort out the many possible causes and plan a course of treatment. Americans spend over $750 million each year on medications and therapies for constipation. Many people believe they must have a bowel movement every day, but there is no evidence that daily bowel movements are necessary. Stool, or feces, is made up of food particles that cannot be absorbed. While these particles contain wastes that are no longer needed by the body, they are not toxic. Constipation is the most common digestive complaint in the United States. It is generally not a serious medical problem. You can usually prevent problems by eating a high-fiber diet as outlined in the Dakota Diet, drinking more fluids, exercising regularly, and allow yourself plenty of time to go to the bathroom.

FRUITS AND VEGETABLES RICH IN ANTIOXIDANTS AND PHYTONUTRIENTS

Research supports the notion that the nutrient value of eating whole foods results in fewer cancers and a decreased risk of heart disease. Ongoing research by scientists in universities worldwide is attempting to identify the exact elements in these foods that are responsible for preventing disease. We have known of the health benefits of fiber for years and are just beginning to realize the health benefits of consuming foods—particularly fruits and vegetables—rich in antioxidants and other phytonutrients (plant nutrients).

Antioxidants include vitamins A, C, and E as well as trace minerals such as selenium and zinc. They work against the oxidative process, which causes cellular damage. Oxidation of cells is the reason why a banana eventually turns brown or apple slices yellow after they have been exposed to the air. The cells within our own body can undergo similar oxidation and become damaged in much the same way. Cellular damage occurs as a result of the formation of free radicals within the cell—highly reactive molecules that begin to damage surrounding structures such as DNA or even the cell membrane. Free radicals can be of some benefit, especially when they are used by the immune system to kill invading bacteria, but excessive amounts can damage the cell and its contents.

Free radicals are formed when an atom interacts with oxygen, causing it to lose one of its orbiting electrons. These molecules (group of atoms) with an odd or unpaired electron try to steal another electron from the nearest molecule, making it a free radical. This chain reaction results in the death of the living cell and the development of a number of diseases, including cancer and heart disease.

The body defends itself by the production of antioxidants, which neutralize free radicals by donating one of their electrons, stopping this chain of events before the cell becomes damaged. The body cannot manufacture antioxidants, so we must obtain them through the diet. The foods of the Dakotas are packed with these vital phytonutrients: fruits, vegetables, nuts, whole grains, and range-fed cattle, buffalo, and wild game feature a full spectrum of vitamins such as C and E as well as selenium, zinc, flavonoids, and carotenoids.

Vitamin E is one of the chief antioxidants. The National Institutes of Health (NIH) has shown that taking up to 200 IU (international units) of vitamin E can provide some benefit in prostate cancer, and other studies have shown vitamin E aids in protecting against Alzheimer's disease, cataracts, and cellular damage from free radicals. Vitamin C (ascorbic acid) is probably the most well-known and studied of all the vitamins. Not only is it a potent antioxidant, it can help improve iron absorption in the stomach as well as regenerate the vitamin E supplies in your body. Because it is water-soluble, vitamin C is not known to cause toxicity in high doses.

Unless you're on a fast food diet and continue to eat poorly, I would not recommend that you stock your medicine cabinet with mega-doses of vitamins as more is not necessarily helpful. The long-term effect of large doses of antioxidants has yet to be proven. The scientific community agrees, however, that eating adequate amounts of fruits and vegetables can lower your risk for developing heart disease and certain cancers. The best advice I can offer is to get your daily dose of antioxidants by eating five to eight servings of whole fruits and vegetables per day.

Antioxidants

Vitamin C

Vitamin C protects cells from damage by free radicals and almost every cell in the body needs it. Vitamin C is a water-soluble vitamin that can only be obtained through diet. Heart disease, cancer, skin disease, and gum disease have all been linked to vitamin C deficiencies. Vitamin C can be found in fruits and vegetables such as strawberries, parsley, broccoli, bell pepper, cauliflower, kale, mustard greens, and Brussels sprouts.

Vitamin E

Vitamin E helps the body neutralize free radicals and also protects the skin from the damaging effects of ultraviolet light. Vitamin E is a family of nutrients with at least eight different structural elements that have different protective properties. Members of the vitamin E family include tocopherols and tocotrienols. For example, the vitamin E used in supplements is alpha-tocopherol, but research has shown that it is the gamma-tocopherols that inhibit cancer of the prostate. Foods rich in vitamin E can help reduce the incidence of bladder cancer. Research has also shown that vitamin E from foods rather than supplements is protective against Alzheimer's disease. Additional research suggests that higher doses of vitamin E could cause harm in the ill or the elderly. Excellent sources of vitamin E include mustard greens, chard, sunflower seeds, turnip greens, and spinach.

Carotenoids

Carotenoids are potent antioxidants that have been shown to stop the damage of free radicals on cellular structures. The color of fruits and vegetables are determined by the type of carotenoid they contain.

Beta-carotene is the reason for yellow and orange colors. Vitamin A is a fat-soluble retinol and is derived from the carotenoid family (beta-carotene, alpha-carotene, and gamma-carotene). It bolsters the immune system and helps with night vision. You can increase your intake of vitamin A or beta-carotene by eating more red and yellow vegetables such as sweet potatoes, carrots, kale, winter squash, and collard greens. Signs of vitamin A deficiency include brittle finger nails, fatigue, loss of the sense of smell, and appetite loss. However, excess vitamin A obtained though supplements can increase your risk for osteoporosis.

Lycopene is responsible for the coloring of red fruits and vegetables, such as tomatoes, grapefruit, and watermelons. Lycopene is considered the most potent antioxidant of all the carotenoids. Eating foods rich in lycopene may reduce the risk of developing prostate cancer. Studies suggest that men should eat at least five servings a week of lycopene-rich foods, such as tomatoes, rather then taking supplements to ward off prostate cancer.

Lutein is the carotenoid that makes foods yellow and green. This carotenoid accumulates in the yellow spot of the retina, where visual perception is most acute. Eating foods rich in lutein can help fight age-related macular degeneration. Lutein can be found in eggs, kale, spinach, turnip greens, collard greens, romaine lettuce, broccoli, zucchini, peas, and Brussels sprouts.

Flavonoids

It is called the "French paradox": research suggests that the French population has a reduced risk for developing heart disease, even though the French diet is higher in saturated fat than most other countries. Their lower rate of heart disease may be due to their love for red wine. Studies have found that wine contains potent antioxidants known as flavonoids, which are found in the seeds and skins of grapes. Flavonoids are a type of pigment that gives many other fruits and vegetables their red and purple colors. Sources of flavonoids include apples, blueberries, pears, raspberries, strawberries, black beans, cabbage, onions, parsley, pinto beans, and tomatoes. Even cocoa beans contain flavonoids—that's why eating dark chocolate is better for your cholesterol than eating regular chocolate. Ongoing research has shown that those who eat flavonoid-enriched foods were 32% less likely to suffer from heart disease and strokes. They have also been shown to reduce blood clots as well as prevent cholesterol from damaging blood vessels.

Selenium

Selenium is a trace element found in varying amounts in foods such as whole-wheat bread, oats, orange juice, and turnips. Studies have shown that consuming foods with adequate amounts of selenium lowers your risk of developing cancers of the lung, colon, bladder, rectum, breast, pancreas, and ovary. Additionally, experts from the American Cancer Society believe that selenium may reduce the risk of prostate cancer by as much as 60%.

Phytonutrients

B-Complex Vitamins

Vitamin B_1 (thiamin) helps the body convert carbohydrates into energy and is important for proper functioning of the heart and nervous systems. We sometimes see thiamin deficiency in older adults as well as alcoholics. Vitamin B_1 can be found in asparagus, mushrooms, spinach, sunflower seeds, lentils, tomatoes, asparagus, and Brussels sprouts.

Vitamin B_2 (riboflavin) helps red blood cells carry oxygen better and boosts the immune system to fight infections. It aids in tissue repair by helping to speed wound healing after burns or other injuries. Riboflavin also works as an antioxidant, preventing free radical damage to cells that help protect the eye's lens from forming cataracts. Excellent sources of vitamin B_2 are mushrooms, spinach, venison, soybeans, beef, and buffalo.

Vitamin B_3 (niacin) is often recommended by physicians as a supplement to help lower cholesterol in the body. It not only lowers total cholesterol but also raises the good (HDL) cholesterol while lowering the bad (LDL) cholesterol. It aids in many other functions in the body, such as the digestive and nervous systems. Good sources include salmon, chicken breast, lamb, venison, turkey, and asparagus.

Vitamin B_5 (pantothenic acid), like vitamin B_2, helps the body convert carbohydrates into energy and may help to lower overall cholesterol levels while raising HDL cholesterol. Deficiencies of this vitamin are rare in humans due to the fact that there are many foods that contain it. Mushrooms are an excellent food source of vitamin B_5 and cauliflower is another good source. Other good sources include eggs, strawberries, broccoli, turnip greens, and sunflower seeds.

Vitamin B_6 (pyridoxine) helps protect against heart problems by lowering levels of homocysteine in the body, an amino acid associated with cardiovascular disease. It aids in the production of important amino acids that are the building blocks of proteins in the body. Vitamin B_6 also plays a role in keeping our immune system functioning properly. Vitamin B_6 can be found in bell peppers, spinach, turkey, salmon, and beef or buffalo.

Vitamin B_{12} (cobalamin), along with vitamins B_6 and folic acid, helps to reduce homocysteine levels. It also helps red blood cells work properly and maintains the fatty substance around the nerve known as the myelin sheath. A deficiency can cause nerve damage resulting in numbness, tingling sensations in the hands and feet, and fatigue. Deficiencies in this vitamin are seen in the elderly as well as vegetarians and those with absorption problems (as seen in Crohn's disease). There may be a potential benefit in treating the effects of aging as well as Alzheimer's disease with a monthly B_{12} shot from your physician. Salmon, beef, lamb, buffalo, venison, and wild game are good sources of vitamin B_{12}.

Folic Acid

Folic acid helps lower homocysteine levels in the body, which in turn helps prevent damage to the lining of blood vessels and plaque build-up. Research also suggests that low levels of this important vitamin may contribute to the development of Alzheimer's disease. Folic acid is also very important for healthy fetal development, especially during the first three months of pregnancy. Deficiencies may place the developing fetus at risk for birth defects of the spinal cord. Because this vitamin is water-soluble, what the body does not use is eliminated in the urine, so deficiencies can occur if your diet is lacking. Physicians recommend that pregnant mothers take supplements in order to reduce the chance of serious birth defects. Excellent sources of folate include romaine lettuce, spinach, asparagus, turnip greens, collard greens, broccoli, cauliflower, beets, and lentils.

PROTEIN

Protein is a macronutrient that your body uses as building blocks for structures such as muscles and hemoglobin (the part of the red blood cell that carries oxygen to the cells). When you eat foods that contain protein, the digestive tract breaks them down into very basic units known as amino acids. The stomach and small intestine quickly absorb these smaller macronutrients to be reused and reassembled into the proteins your body needs to keep muscles, blood, body organs, bones, and the immune system healthy.

There are 22 different types of amino acids that are important to human health. The body can make only 13 of them, with the rest considered to be "essential" amino acids because they can only be obtained from the diet.

The proteins from animal sources contain all nine essential amino acids that the body needs. Vegetable proteins can be incomplete because they lack some of the essential amino acids the body needs for good health. Vegetarians can still get all of their essential amino acids by eating a wide variety of vegetables.

This chapter has presented our new understanding of what constitutes good nutrition, with a particular emphasis on good and bad fats. It turns out that the original diet of the Plains Indians of the Dakotas is one we should learn to emulate, according to modern science. We will now look at specific foods in the Dakota Diet and how they can become a vital part of your healthy eating plan.

CHAPTER 3

Healthy Foods from the Dakotas

N ow that we've reviewed some general guidelines on good nutrition, we can take a look at the foods in the Dakota Diet that can help you get the nutrients you need to stay healthy and prevent disease. Fortunately, today, we have access to a wide range of healthy foods, common in the Dakotas and across America. These fruits, vegetables and legumes, grains, nuts, and proteins provide all the nutrition necessary for a vibrant life and, if eaten in accordance with the Dakota Diet, can also help you lose excess weight at the same time.

EAT YOUR FRUITS AND VEGETABLES

The National Institutes of Health (NIH) recommends consuming at least five servings of fruits and vegetables a day. There are many reasons to do this, and one is that most fruits (and some vegetables) can be eaten right on the spot—nature's fast food, so to speak. They require little or no preparation. Why is it, then, that many Americans are not getting enough of these vital foods in the diet? Many feel that fresh foods cost too much, but the reality is that the nutritional value of fresh fruits and vegetables far exceeds the monetary value. One way to reduce your cost is to buy foods in season, which are typically cheaper and have a better taste because they are harvested at their prime.

Eat a variety of fruits and vegetables in order to get all the necessary nutrients, such as calcium, iron, and vitamin C. You will increase your likelihood of getting adequate nutritional value by varying the foods you eat. Remember, you are on a diet, so eating fried foods such as french fries or chips does not count as a vegetable.

Many people are concerned about harmful pesticides used to protect crops from insects and molds. Our fruit and vegetable supply does not contain excessive pesticide residues, according to the U.S. Food and Drug Administration (FDA), which is responsible for monitoring pesticides in our foods. The benefit of eating whole foods far outweighs any risk of pesticide exposure. Some health food stores have fruits and vegetables grown organically, without pesticides, which may cost a bit more, but the nutrient value will justify the expense.

Removing Pesticides From Fruits and Vegetables

If you are concerned about pesticides, take these steps to protect yourself:

1. Wash fruits and vegetables with water and a scrub brush before eating them.

2. Peel and cook, when appropriate.

3. Peel away the outer layer of a leafy vegetable, such as lettuce and cabbage.

FRUITS OF THE DAKOTAS

The main sugar in fruit is called fructose—fruit's natural sweetener, so to speak. It is a simple sugar but one that is broken down slowly when the whole fruit is eaten. The amount of fructose in a fruit depends on the type of fruit and where it is produced. Sweeter tasting fruit typically has more simple sugar in it. Fruit in areas of the world with longer growing seasons will be sweeter than fruit grown in areas with shorter seasons. Most of the fruits from the Midwest may not be as sweet tasting but are loaded with phytonutrients that can benefit your health.

The fiber in fruit helps keep blood sugar levels stable. This fiber, called pectin, is a water-soluble colloidal carbohydrate (polysaccharide) present in ripe fruit. Fruits high in pectin include peaches, apples, and plums. Pectin is an indigestible soluble fiber and functions as an intestinal regulator.

> Fresh fruit: Eat five a day to help keep the doctor away.

The color of the fruit is a good indicator as to the phytonutrient the fruit contains. For example, red fruits such as tomatoes and watermelon typically contain lycopene. Red, purple, and orange indicates ellagic acid, quercetin, and resveratrol, respectively—found in strawberries, grapes, raspberries, and cantaloupe.

Apples

My fondest childhood memories were of the days when my mother would allow us to harvest the apples from the trees in our neighborhood to make apple pie. The apple is a low-calorie fruit loaded with fiber and phytonutrients. It contains both soluble and insoluble fiber: a medium-sized apple can contain up to 3 grams of fiber. Insoluble fiber prevents the absorption of cholesterol in the digestive tract and soluble fiber (pectin) helps to reduce the amount of LDL (bad) cholesterol produced by the liver. Fiber also helps to relieve constipation, preventing diverticulosis and even colon cancer.

Apples also contain antioxidants that help neutralize free radicals, thus preventing oxidative damage and cell death. In fact, one apple has as much antioxidant activity as 1,500 mg of vitamin C. Flavonoids are another reason why you should eat an apple a day. Research has shown that those who ate foods rich in flavonoids had at least a 20% reduction in heart disease. The apple's pigment (color) is the main source of these cholesterol-lowering flavonoids, which also help to prevent the oxidation of LDL cholesterol.

Blueberries

Blueberries are another low-calorie fruit loaded with antioxidants to help destroy free radicals. Anthocyanidins are the primary phytonutrient in blueberries, responsible for their blue pigment, and found to help prevent heart disease. Wine, especially red wine, is another good source of anthocyanidins. A recent study found that blueberries have almost 40% more of these cardioprotective antioxidants than wine. Another potent antioxidant found in blueberries, known as pterostilbene, has been shown to reduce heart disease by helping the liver metabolize cholesterol. Blueberries are high in soluble fiber (pectin), which helps to lower cholesterol and fight cancer.

Cantaloupe

Cantaloupe is in the same family as squash and cucumbers. Many back yard gardens can support this low-calorie melon packed with nutrients. It is an excellent source of beta-carotene, which the body converts to vitamin A. One cup of cantaloupe has only 56 calories and over 100% of the recommended dietary allowance (RDA) of vitamin A. Vitamin A is a powerful fat-soluble antioxidant that can protect the eyes from cataracts, improve night vision, and prevent macular degeneration. Cantaloupe is also rich in vitamin C. Both of these potent antioxidants help prevent free radical damage as well as boost the immune system.

Pears

Pears are related to the apple and are a good source of vitamin C and copper. Both are antioxidants that help protect the body from the damaging effects of free radicals. The fiber in pears helps bind cancer-causing chemicals in the colon as well as lower cholesterol by binding to bile salts that are made from cholesterol. Pears are a hypoallergenic fruit, a safe fruit to introduce to infants. The pear season in the Midwest runs from August to October, but pears can be found year round in grocery stores.

Plums

Another seasonal fruit found in much of the Midwest is the plum. There are many varieties of plums that can be found not only in the wild, but also at your local cooperative or grocery store. Dried plums are known as prunes, a favorite for those suffering from constipation. Plums contain phenols (neochlorogenic and cholorogenic acid), which are potent antioxidants that help prevent the oxidation of cholesterol circulating in the blood. They also are a good source of vitamin C, vitamin E, beta-carotene, vitamin B_2, and fiber.

Raspberries

Ellagic acid is a substance found in raspberries that is responsible for most of this fruit's antioxidant activity. Raspberries also contain other flavonoids with potent antioxidant properties that may have anti-cancer potential. They are rich in vitamin C and are a good source of riboflavin, folate, niacin, and copper. They also contain soluble fiber in the form of pectin, which lowers cholesterol.

Rhubarb

Rhubarb is a perennial plant that grows from rhizomes. The stem of the plant is usually cooked and sweetened for pies and cakes, but it can be eaten raw. Rhubarb stems are rich in anthraquinones, which are cathartic and laxative. This explains its use as a laxative when eaten in large quantities. Rhubarb also contains calcium, vitamin K, and lutein.

Strawberries

Strawberries are at their peak in the early summer months, but most varieties can be found in your local grocery store year round and are an excellent source of vitamin C, vitamin K, and manganese. Other nutrients include folate and copper as well as omega-3 fatty acids. They also have very potent antioxidants in the form of phenols, which have been shown to have anti-inflammatory as well as anti-cancer properties.

Watermelon

Believe it or not, watermelon is an excellent source of vitamin C and lycopene, which has been studied extensively and is proven to be protective against breast, prostate, lung, and colon cancers. Watermelon is also rich in B vitamins, which can lower the risk for heart disease. It has a higher water content and lower calorie count than most other fruits on the market. I consider this a nutrient-dense fruit that delivers more nutrients than calories.

VEGETABLES OF THE DAKOTAS

Remember as a child having your mother remind you to "eat your vegetables"? She was right, of course. Even the U.S. Department of Health and Human Services acknowledges what our mothers already knew—eating vegetables can have many health benefits. If only our government leaders had listened to their own mothers on health and nutrition, then perhaps we would not have such an obesity epidemic in this country. The health benefits of eating vegetables cannot be overstated. Most of the produce grown in the Midwest is loaded with flavor and nutrients. Just like the fruits of the Dakotas, the color of the vegetable can tell you what type of phytonutrients it contains.

Many gardens of the Dakotas and across the United States can support a variety of vegetables. The reward of gardening goes beyond eating a healthy product that's low in calories and loaded with nutrients—it can also increase your bone density. A study compared the bone density of women who do aerobics to women who garden and found that gardeners have higher bone density, as the work they do is weight-bearing and also keeps them in the sun, which provides them with vitamin D.

Asparagus

Asparagus is a succulent and tender vegetable that has a growing season in the Midwest from early spring through July, but it is often available for longer periods in grocery stores. It is an excellent source of folate, which helps lower homocysteine levels in the blood. One serving of asparagus (1 cup or 3–4 spears) can supply up to 60% of the RDA of folate. Along with folate, asparagus contains the immune-building minerals zinc and selenium as well as vitamin C.

Homocysteine

Homocysteine is an amino acid found in the blood. Epidemiological studies have indicated that too much homocysteine in the blood is related to a higher risk of heart disease. However, a direct causal link has not been established yet, according to the American Heart Association.

Bell Peppers

Whether the pepper is green, yellow, red, or orange, this highly nutritious vegetable is rich in vitamins C and A. These two powerful antioxidants help reduce the effects of free radicals responsible for causing damage to cells as well as the build up of cholesterol in the arteries. Vitamin A has also been shown to reduce the incidence of lung cancer. A study published in *Cancer Epidemiology, Biomarkers and Prevention* showed a very low rate of lung disease, including cancer, in adults eating foods rich in vitamin A. Red bell peppers are rich in lycopene, a carotenoid that has been shown to reduce the incidence of cancer of the prostate, cervix, bladder, and pancreas. Bell peppers are also rich in another carotenoid, beta-cryptoxanthin, that has produced a 37% reduction in the risk of lung cancer in smokers when compared to smokers who did not eat bell peppers.

Broccoli

Broccoli, a member of the cabbage family, is available in most grocery stores year round. Broccoli contains phytochemicals called sulforaphane and indoles. Indoles have been shown to suppress breast tumor growth, and sulforaphane boosts the immune system's ability to remove cancer-causing substances. Studies by the American Cancer Society have recognized indoles as a promising anti-cancer agent that attacks reproductive tumor cells, including cancers of the prostate gland in men. Broccoli also contains folate and other B vitamins that help lower homocysteine in the blood. It has the RDA for vitamin C in one serving as well as small amounts of zinc and selenium, helping to boost your immune system.

Brussels Sprouts

Brussels sprouts are closely related to cabbage and available year round in almost any grocery store. Brussels sprouts are high in vitamin C, folate (folic acid), and other phytochemicals that help the body fight disease. If you want to increase the fiber in your diet, one cup of these little cabbages will add up to 4 grams of fiber, which will promote a healthy colon and even help prevent heart disease by blocking the absorption of cholesterol in your diet.

Cabbage

Cabbage is rich in vitamin C and a good source of fiber for colon health and heart disease prevention. A study published in the *Journal of Cancer Research* demonstrated a reduction in breast cancer in women who eat more of the Brassica family of vegetables (broccoli, cabbage, cauliflower, kale, and Brussels sprouts). Another study showed a reduction in colon cancer as well.

Cauliflower

Most of the Brassica family of vegetables, including cauliflower, contain vitamin C. They also contain a sulfur-like compound that, when digested, aids in the liver's response to detoxify cancer-causing substances (carcinogens).

Celery

Celery contains coumarins, which help prevent free radicals from damaging cells and they also help white blood cells do a better job in targeting and eliminating harmful agents. Celery will also lower blood pressure as a result of active compounds called phthalides, which relax muscles of the arteries and allowing the vessel to dilate (in much the same way as the pharmaceutical nitrates affect blood pressure). Animal studies showed a blood pressure reduction of 14% when injected with a small dose of phthalide (equivalent to roughly four stalks of celery for humans).

Collard Greens

Traditionally recognized as a staple of the South, collard greens can be grown in just about any soil and are available year round. The health benefits include phytonutrients with anti-cancer properties to help detoxify carcinogens. The main antioxidants in collard greens are vitamin C, vitamin E, and beta-carotene. The calcium found in collard greens can help maintain strong bones and even reduce colon cancer by neutralizing cancer-causing chemicals. Collard greens are a good source of heart-protective B vitamins as well as potassium and magnesium, which have been shown to lower blood pressure. The fiber contained in collard greens can also lower your cholesterol and prevent constipation. Collard greens also contain omega-3 fatty acids as well as iron and protein, making this an excellent dietary choice to either plant in your garden or buy at your local grocery store.

Cucumber

The cucumber is primarily composed of water but is also rich in fiber and minerals such as silica, magnesium, and potassium. Silica promotes healthy connective tissue and may improve one's complexion. The Dietary Approaches to Stop Hypertension (DASH) study showed a reduction in blood pressure among those who ate a diet rich in potassium, magnesium, and fiber.

Eggplant

Eggplant contains a variety of vitamins and minerals as well as other phytonutrients with antioxidant properties. Research from the U.S. Department of Agriculture has shown that eggplant is a rich source of phenolic compounds such as nasunin, which protects against damage to cell membranes. Eggplant also contains cholorogenic acid, a potent free radical scavenger that can help fight cancer as well as lower your LDL (bad) cholesterol. It is also low in calories and high in fiber and contains other B vitamins proven to lower homocysteine levels.

Garlic

Garlic is a bulb that can be grown in many areas throughout the Midwest and other parts of the U.S. This popular spice can add flavor to many dishes and its health benefits are well documented. A member of the Allium family, garlic is an excellent source of manganese, vitamin B_6, vitamin C, and selenium. Studies have shown that garlic can lower blood pressure and LDL (bad) cholesterol while raising HDL (good) cholesterol in the blood. A 2004 study in *Preventive Medicine* showed that garlic can also prevent plaque formation in the arteries by inhibiting calcification of coronary arteries.

Green Beans

Green beans (or string beans) are an excellent source of vitamin C as well as fiber and beta-carotene. These are important antioxidants that prevent the oxidation of cholesterol, lessening the likelihood of plaque build-up within the arteries. These antioxidants also prevent colon cancer by protecting the cells from damage when they are exposed to other cancer-causing agents. The fiber in green beans helps bind carcinogens in the diet, such as nitrosamines, thus ridding the body of these toxins before they cause harm to the colon.

Green Peas

Green peas are a good source of vitamin K, which helps with bone density by activating osteocalcin, a protein that maintains the calcium levels inside the bone. Green peas are rich in vitamin B_6 and folic acid, both of which help lower homocysteine levels in the blood. Homocysteine can not only cause atherosclerosis, it can also weaken the bone matrix, resulting in osteoporosis. Green peas are also a great source of vitamins B_1 (thiamine), B_2 (riboflavin), B_3 (niacin), and B_6, all essential in the metabolism of carbohydrates, protein, and fat. Peas also contain vitamin C, which has anti-cancer properties and protects the cells' DNA from damage.

Kale

Kale is a member of the cabbage family and can be cultivated in most gardens. It is excellent when sautéed with fresh garlic and sprinkled with lemon juice and olive oil. It is also great on homemade pizza. Kale is loaded with vitamin A and lutein, which have been shown to reduce the risk of cataracts. Kale contains other nutrients such as vitamin C and the B vitamins, which have been shown to reduce the risk for heart disease and cancer. Kale is a good source of fiber and calcium, making this a good choice for a healthy colon and strong bones.

Leeks

Leeks are of the Allium family, just like garlic and onions. They can be found in the grocery store all year long and are a bit sweeter than onions. A diet high in Allium vegetables helps lower LDL (bad) and total cholesterol as well as raise HDL (good) cholesterol levels in the body. Research has also proven that a diet including these types of vegetables two or more times a week can reduce the risk of prostate and colon cancers. Leeks and other Allium vegetables help slow the absorption of sugars in the intestine, which will help stabilize blood sugar levels in the body.

Onions

The health benefits of eating onions include lowering cholesterol and blood pressure. Onions are rich in chromium, which reduces heart disease by lowering cholesterol and triglyceride levels in the body. Chromium has also been shown to decrease blood glucose levels by competing with insulin in the liver, where insulin is inactivated—this allows more insulin to be available at the cellular level. Studies have also shown that eating onions and other members of the Allium family (like garlic) can significantly reduce the risk of developing colon cancer.

Parsley

Even though parsley is native to the Mediterranean culture, this leafy spice can be grown in just about any garden. Its major role is as a table garnish, but I would not ignore its nutritional value. Parsley contains an oil called myristicin, which has been shown to inhibit the formation of tumor cells. The flavonoids in parsley include luteolin, another potent antioxidant that helps to prevent damage to cells. Parsley is an excellent source of three nutrients that are vital for the prevention of disease: vitamin C, beta-carotene, and folic acid.

Romaine Lettuce

Eating lettuce before a meal is a great way to eat a high–water volume food, low in calories and packed with nutrients. Start your meal with a salad and enjoy the benefits of eating a food that is an excellent source of vitamins A and C, folate, and plentiful antioxidants. Romaine lettuce can be grown fairly easily in most soils. It can be purchased fresh all year long in most grocery stores.

Spinach

Even Popeye knew the benefits of eating spinach. Spinach has a number of flavonoids that function as antioxidants, which can prevent cancer, including colon and prostate cancers. Spinach also contains lutein, a carotenoid that can slow macular degeneration in some people, and neoxanthin, a carotenoid that has been shown to help kill off prostate cancer cells and prevent further growth. Spinach can give you strong bones, lower homocysteine levels as a result of its folic acid content, and prevent heart disease with the power of antioxidants like vitamin A and C. The amount of iron in cooked spinach compares to red meat, with fewer calories. Eating spinach with vitamin C–rich foods, such as tomatoes or citrus fruits, will increase the absorption of this mineral.

Summer Squash

This hardy vegetable is a favorite for many gardeners and is available throughout the year. Though research on its phytonutrients is limited, squash is considered to have the same anti-cancer effects attributed to many of the root vegetables. Squash is an excellent source of vitamins C and A, fiber, folate, and copper. All have been shown to reduce heart disease by lowering cholesterol and preventing the oxidation of cholesterol, which reduces plaque build-up in the arteries.

Tomato

In a botanical sense, the tomato is actually a fruit, and arguably has been studied more than any other food for its health benefits. Tomatoes are loaded with lycopene, which has been shown to protect against colon, prostate, breast, lung, and pancreatic cancers. Tomatoes are also loaded with other vital phytonutrients with antioxidant properties that help protect against cancer and heart disease. Tomatoes are a good source of fiber, which has been shown to lower cholesterol levels and prevent colon cancer as well.

Turnip Greens

Turnip greens are an excellent source of vitamins A, C, and E, as well as calcium and the B vitamins. This vegetable has an amazing combination of antioxidants that can prevent cancer and slow the progression of heart disease.

Winter Squash

The phytonutrient value of winter squash is just beginning to be understood. There are many varieties of this hardy food, once an important part of the Native Americans' diet. Winter squash is loaded with vitamin A, shown to lower the risk for lung cancer in smokers and to improve the symptoms of emphysema. Along with vitamin A (beta-carotene), squash is abundant in vitamins C, B_1, B_3, and B_6, which are heart protective by lowering cholesterol. Protection against lung and heart disease are not the only benefits: studies have shown that eating foods like winter squash that are rich in beta-carotene can also protect the colon from damage by cancer-causing chemicals. Folate is also found in winter squash—it can lower homocysteine levels and even prevents certain birth defects in children.

ROOT VEGETABLES AND LEGUMES OF THE DAKOTAS

Root vegetables are plant parts that store energy underground in the form of carbohydrates. They include true roots and taproots, as well as non-roots such as tubers, rhizomes, corms, and bulbs.

Legumes (beans and lentils) come from plants with edible pods. Legumes are a good source of fiber and phytonutrients crucial to a healthy diet. The dietary fiber in legumes provides many health benefits, such as controlling blood sugar levels and lowering cholesterol. The high fiber content of legumes helps to slow the absorption of simple sugars in the diet, which prevents sugars in the blood from rising too rapidly, making legumes a great food choice for the natural control of diabetes. The fiber in legumes also binds bile acids responsible for the production of cholesterol. Because the fiber is not absorbed, it exits the body, taking bile acids with it.

Legumes are a good source of iron, an important component of hemoglobin. Hemoglobin in the blood is responsible for transporting oxygen from the lungs to the cells in the body. Having adequate iron stores is important for this process to occur. Women who menstruate may become iron deficient, so eating plenty of legumes is especially important. One cup of any type of legume will give you up to 30% of the RDA of iron.

If you are a vegetarian, legumes are a good source of protein without the saturated fat found in processed meats. One cup will typically provide up to 15 grams of protein or 30% of the RDA. Legumes also contain a number of antioxidants, such as thiamine (vitamin B_1), which helps improve memory. A lack of thiamine in the body has been shown to contribute to age-related decline in memory as seen in Alzheimer's disease. One cup of legumes will provide you with 19% of the RDA for thiamine.

Root Vegetables

Beets

Beets are crunchy and sweet, with the highest sugar content of all vegetables, yet low in calories. Betacyanin is the pigment that gives beets their rich color and is a phytonutrient with cancer-fighting properties. Studies have shown that beets protect against heart disease by lowering LDL (bad) cholesterol and triglyceride levels in the blood and raising HDL (good) cholesterol.

Beets are rich in the B vitamin folate, which can prevent certain birth defects when taken during pregnancy. The RDA for folate is 400 micrograms (mcg). Just one cup of boiled, sliced beets contains 136 mcg of folate, or 34% of the dietary requirement.

Carrots

Carrots are loaded with carotenoids, which convert to vitamin A in the body. A diet rich in these phytonutrients helps protect against heart disease and cancer. Vitamin A improves night vision and protects against macular degeneration. The anti-cancer properties of carotenoids have been studied extensively and include a significant reduction in cancers of the bladder, colon, cervix, and prostate. Smokers will benefit from a diet high in carotenoids as studies have shown a reduction in lung cancer and emphysema.

Horseradish

Horseradish is a root that can be harvested twice a year, even in the Dakotas. It is a member of the mustard family and related to cabbage, cauliflower, Brussels sprouts, and the common radish. It is not hot until its volatile oils, known as isothiocyanates, are released when grated. Vinegar stops this process (the sooner vinegar is added, the milder the final product).

One tablespoonful of horseradish has 6 calories, 1.4 grams of carbohydrate, and no fat. It also contains sodium, potassium, calcium, and phosphorus. Because horseradish has so much flavor and no fat, the National Heart, Lung, and Blood Institute has recommended it as a substitute for other condiments. Horseradish can be added to eggs before cooking, as a topping for cooked vegetables instead of butter, and mixed with other condiments to add flavor and reduce fat.

Sweet Potatoes

The sweet potato is a traditional Thanksgiving treat, but it can be enjoyed throughout the year. Its yellowish-orange flesh is often confused with the yam. They are unique in flavor and texture, yet have many similar health benefits that have been extensively researched. Some scientists have described the sweet potato as an anti-diabetic food in that it can stabilize blood sugar levels and lower insulin resistance. The sweet potato has potent antioxidants, such as vitamin A and vitamin C, and is also a good source of fiber, potassium, and copper.

Yams

Often confused with the sweet potato, the yam is available throughout the year as well. Yams are an excellent source of vitamin B_6, which helps lower homocysteine levels in the body. Yams are also a good source of potassium, which has been shown to lower blood pressure. They are loaded with fiber and complex carbohydrates to help control blood sugar levels and lower insulin resistance.

Legumes

Black Beans

Black beans are rich in antioxidants such as anthocyanidins, the chief antioxidant found in many fruits. Black beans also contain folate, which helps to lower homocysteine levels in the blood. Magnesium is another benefit of eating black beans. This trace mineral is known to lower blood pressure, a risk factor for heart disease. One cup of black beans will provide you with up to 60% of the RDA of folate and 30% of the RDA of magnesium.

Dried Peas

Peas contain phytonutrients such as isoflavones, which have been shown to reduce the incidence of hormonally sensitive cancers, such as breast and prostate cancer.

Kidney Beans

Like many of the legumes, kidney beans are a rich source of both folate and magnesium, nutrients that help protect the heart by lowering both homocysteine levels in the blood and blood pressure.

Lentils

Lentils are easy to prepare, are available throughout the year, and are a great source of fiber and phytonutrients. Lentils are good for the heart and the bowels, thanks in part to their healthy dose of insoluble fiber.

Navy Beans

These white beans were once the staple food on U.S. naval ships and can be found year-round in most stores. They are a good source of fiber and protein along with other nutrients such as thiamine, copper, magnesium, and iron.

Pinto Beans

Pinto beans are colorful and, like other beans, loaded with fiber and phytonutrients. They can be found either dried or canned throughout the year. Much like lentils, eating pinto beans will provide you with many similar health benefits.

NUTS OF THE DAKOTAS

It's okay to go nuts over nuts, but don't overdo it. Nuts are loaded with heart-healthy monounsaturated fats as well as fiber and phytonutrients. The key in eating them, however, is portion control, because 1 ounce of nuts can have as many as 200 calories.

Numerous studies have shown the health benefits of eating nuts. They not only contain fiber and monounsaturated fats, but also vitamin E and copper. One ounce of nuts per day can help lower LDL (bad) cholesterol and raise HDL (good) cholesterol. The fiber in nuts has also been shown to lower total cholesterol in the body.

I have made a list of some common nuts and seeds found on the plains of the Dakotas and in most grocery stores. Just about any nut can be used as a nutritious filler, but remember to keep your portions small and avoid snack bags of nuts, as the manufacturers generally load these with flavorings and partially hydrogenated oils (trans-fats).

Pumpkin Seeds

Pumpkins are in the same vegetable family as cucumber and squash. The seeds contain cucurbitacins, which prevent the body from converting testosterone to the more potent dihydrotestosterone (DHT) form. This can help avoid prostate enlargement in men. Pumpkin seeds also contain zinc, which aids the immune system and helps to fight off viruses such as the common cold. Zinc can also help prevent the development of osteoporosis in both men and women. Other minerals such as magnesium, phosphorus, and manganese are found in pumpkin seeds. They are also a good source of iron, copper, protein, and monounsaturated fats.

Sunflower Seeds

Sunflower seeds have a wealth of nutrition: they are very high in polyunsaturated oils and are loaded with vitamin E, magnesium, and selenium. Vitamin E is a fat-soluble antioxidant that neutralizes free radicals in the body. In the prevention of cardiovascular disease, vitamin E prevents free radicals from oxidizing cholesterol (it is the oxidation of cholesterol that causes it to adhere to the walls of blood vessels). Eating $\frac{1}{4}$ cup of sunflower seeds will give you roughly 90% of the RDA of vitamin E. The magnesium in sunflower seeds can reduce blood pressure and promote healthy bones. Selenium is a trace element that has been shown to prevent cancer by repairing DNA in damaged cells as well as by helping the body eliminate damaged or abnormal cells. Selenium also aids other antioxidants by helping the liver detoxify potentially harmful substances.

Walnuts

Walnuts are harvested in the fall but are available throughout the year. This nutritious snack has many health benefits. Walnuts are heart protective because they contain an abundance of omega-3 fats as well as monounsaturated fats. A 2004 study in *Circulation* showed a significant reduction in total cholesterol and LDL (bad) cholesterol related to high blood levels of alpha-linolenic acid (an omega-3 fat) and gamma-tocopherol, a form of vitamin E. Walnuts also have antioxidants that help inhibit free radical damage to LDL cholesterol. Walnuts contain copper and manganese, both important in helping other antioxidants in the defense against cancer. Copper alone has been shown to lower LDL and raise HDL cholesterol.

GRAINS OF THE DAKOTAS

Grains are the seeds of grasses and include wheat, corn, rye, oats, and barley. Each grain contains a seed, or germ, covered by bran and a hull. When the grain is milled and refined, the germ and bran layers are removed in order to shorten the grain's cooking time. Unfortunately, up to 30% of the grain's pro-

Flaxseed: Rich in Omega-3 Fats and Other Anti-Cancer Nutrients

Mahatma Gandhi once said, "Wherever flaxseeds become a regular food item among the people, there will be better health." Flaxseed has been part of the human diet for at least 10,000 years. The seeds, as well as cloth woven from flax, have been found in the ancient tombs of Egypt. No one knows the true origin of flax, as its seeds have been cultivated for many centuries throughout many parts of the world. Flax tends to thrive in both temperate and tropical climates of the world, and it can be found in great quantity on the plains of the Dakotas.

Flaxseed is one of the richest sources of omega-3 fatty acids in the plant world. The benefits of a diet enriched with omega-3 fatty acids cannot be overstated, ranging from cancer prevention to cholesterol reduction to easing inflammation. Flaxseed is approximately 40% oil, with nearly 70% of that oil being omega-3.

Flaxseed is also an abundant source of lignans, a type of insoluble fiber that acts as a phytoestrogen (plant-derived form of estrogen). When phytoestrogens are absorbed, they have a hormonal effect that can relieve many of the symptoms associated with menopause, including hot flashes and mood swings. Additional research suggests that lignans may have anti-cancer properties, which could reduce the rate of breast cancer in women who consume flaxseed. The proof that eating flaxseed will prevent breast cancer is not concrete; however, the evidence for its anti-cancer effect is promising.

tein, much of its B vitamins, and all of its fiber are removed in this process. And even more vitamins are removed when the grain is bleached, turning it into refined white flour.

About one-fifth of the typical American diet consists of foods made from refined wheat in the form of buns, cakes, cookies, and bread. These products lack the nutrients of the whole grain and are usually loaded with fats and simple sugars. When you consume the whole grain, you are eating the germ or seed, which contains essential fats important for health. The hull and bran layers contain protein as well as fiber, B vitamins, and antioxidants. Even

Lignans have received a lot of attention lately for their effect on prostate cancer as well as benign prostatic hypertrophy (BPH or enlarging prostate) in men. Lignans have been shown to block the enzyme that converts testosterone to dihydrotestosterone (DHT), the growth hormone of the prostate. In combination with a low-fat diet, men may be able to relieve many BPH symptoms by consuming at least $\frac{1}{4}$ cup of flax meal a day.

Because most Americans do not get enough fiber or omega-3 fatty acids in their diets, adding flaxseed is a simple and important step toward healthier eating. I recommend having flax meal or seeds on hand at all times. They are inexpensive and can be easily purchased in bulk at any local health food store. Ground flaxseed is preferred to flaxseed oil as it contains lignans as well as omega-3 fatty acids and soluble and insoluble fiber. While you can purchase flax oil rich in omega-3, the amount of lignans will be negligible.

You can grind flaxseed in a coffee bean grinder in order to improve its digestion when eaten. It has a nutty flavor and can be sprinkled on salads, cereal, or yogurt. Ground flaxseed can be added to breads, muffins, waffles, and pancakes as well. It may even help you reduce your appetite before meals as it will absorb approximately eight times its weight in water if taken one hour before a meal.

However, I do not recommend the consumption of more than $\frac{1}{4}$ cup of flaxseed per day as the seeds contain cyanogens. Cyanogens can prevent the thyroid gland from taking up enough iodine, increasing your risk for a goiter.

though the food industry "enriches" refined white breads with B vitamins, white bread still lacks the fiber and protein lost in the milling process.

There are many reasons why you should include whole grains in your diet. Studies have shown that people consuming fiber in whole grains reduce their heart disease risk by as much as 29% when compared to subjects with low fiber intakes. Whole grains are rich in antioxidants, up to 20 times that of refined grains, including vitamin E and selenium, as well as a number of other phytonutrients that prevent the free radical damage of cholesterol. Other benefits of whole grains include phytoestrogens to protect the heart and bones and to prevent hormonally sensitive cancers. Whole grains have potent antioxidants, fiber, and phytonutrients that work as a team in the fight against cancer.

Eat at least three servings of whole grains a day. Have fun experimenting with your favorite recipes or go to your local cooperative or health food store to learn about other ways to incorporate whole grains into your diet.

Barley

Barley puffs up like rice when cooked and has a nutty taste and chewy texture. It is a good source of copper, manganese, fiber, and selenium. One cup of barley can give you up to 50% of the RDA of selenium. Selenium has been shown to lower the incidence of colon cancer, improve the immune system, and aid in thyroid function.

Buckwheat

Buckwheat is actually the seed of a fruit rather than a true grain from grass. It can be consumed as cereal or ground into flour for baking. Buckwheat has a rich supply of flavonoids, which have been shown to protect the heart from disease.

Millet

Millet is a common ingredient in bird seed, but is not necessarily just for the birds. It can be substituted in cooking for rice or other grains. Millet contains magnesium, which has been shown to lower blood pressure, and niacin (vitamin B_3) which helps to lower cholesterol.

Oats

Eating oats can improve heart health by reducing total cholesterol. Oats can also help remove cholesterol by preventing absorption in the digestive system. Antioxidants in oats include selenium, which works with vitamin E in the fight against heart disease as well as reducing the risk for colon cancer. Gluten, a protein found in many grains, causes allergies for many people. Oats, however, have only a small amount of gluten and appear to be better tolerated in those with gluten sensitivity (celiac disease).

Rye

Rye is an excellent source of a non-soluble fiber, which has a high water-binding capacity. This helps in weight loss for the simple reason that you eat less because you feel full sooner when eating rye. Rye also has phytoestrogen activity in the form of lignans, which help to protect against prostate cancer in men and to relieve symptoms of menopause in women.

Wheat

Always remember this—fiber is a carbohydrate. Diets that avoid carbohydrates can result in a number of health problems, such as constipation and diverticulosis. When the whole grain is refined and its fiber is removed, the simple sugars are easily absorbed in the gut causing a sharp rise in blood sugar

> "To love and appreciate the Rocky Mountains, you only open your eyes, but to love and appreciate the prairie, you must open your soul."
>
> –LOUIS TOOTHMAN

levels. Eating whole grains like wheat is important not only for blood sugar control, but it will also provide you with important antioxidants and other phytonutrients important for preventing disease. Wheat contains lignans and other nutrients such as vitamin E that can protect the body from cancers and heart disease. In order to receive this benefit, you have to choose products such as pasta, flour, and breads made from the whole wheat rather than foods made from refined wheat.

MEAT: GRASS-FED MEANS BETTER TASTE AND NUTRITION

I have to admit it—I love to eat meat. There is nothing I enjoy more than to cook a T-bone over an open flame on the grill. Before I began to appreciate the importance of dieting and health, I did not worry about the fat content of meat nor did I pay attention to how the meat was raised or produced.

As I began to research nutrition and health, I started to change my own eating habits. By watching what I ate, I lost weight without a major changes to my lifestyle. Not only did I shed pounds, my LDL (bad) cholesterol levels fell as did my total cholesterol levels, and I was able to raise my HDL (good) cholesterol. I focused on eating nutrient-dense, low-calorie foods such as fresh fruits and vegetables. I avoided fast foods and processed foods high in calories with little nutritional value. I continued to grill my steak, but the meat I cooked was from animals that were allowed to graze on the grasses of the Dakotas, such as buffalo and wild game.

The meat from grass-fed animals has less fat and fewer calories than grain-fed animals. In fact, a 6-ounce steak from a grass-fed animal can have up to 100 fewer calories than a 6-ounce steak from an animal whose diet was mostly grain. Additionally, the amount of omega-3 fat in the meat of grass-fed animals is higher, as is the amount of vitamin E and other nutrients. It is when livestock are sent to the feedlot to be fed a grain-based diet that we see omega-3 fat and other nutrients drastically reduced in the cuts of meat.

Unfortunately, much of the meat produced in this country comes from the feedlot. The food industry prefers this manner because it is relatively inexpensive to fatten the cattle with government-subsidized grain and they are able to produce massive amounts of the product year round.

The price for this cheap food comes at the expense of our health. For example, when cattle are confined in a feedlot, infectious disease can easily spread. To counter this, low-dose antibiotics are mixed in the cattle feed. What has emerged from this indiscriminant use of antibiotics to control bacteria are organisms that are resistant to common drugs such as penicillin. Nearly 70% of all antibiotics made in the United States are used in the cattle industry. Antibiotics are not only used to control disease, they have also been shown to fatten up the livestock before they are sent to slaughter.

Animal waste in the feedlot is another problem. Thousands of cattle are confined in such a way that they are literally living and eating out of their own toilet. When they are sent to slaughter, cleaning the manure off of them can be difficult. A common bacterium known as *E. coli* is found in the manure and can contaminate the meat during the slaughtering process. This bacteria has become acid resistant, meaning that the bacteria can survive in an acidic environment such as our own stomach. Livestock that are able to roam the grasslands live in a cleaner environment and have a much lower risk of contracting diseases common in the feedlot, which in turn are responsible for contaminating the meat during processing.

There is also growing concern among the public over mad cow disease (bovine spongiform encephalopathy or BSE). One theory regarding how cattle contract mad cow disease is the practice of feeding cattle byproduct feed, which includes animal tissue from other cattle. To put it simply, the industry turned herbivores (plant eaters) into carnivores (meat eaters). This risk of BSE is eliminated in cattle raised on the plains of the Dakotas as they are only fed pasture grasses and hay.

Farmers and ranchers are beginning to understand how important it is for their cattle to eat native grasses. Their herds are healthier as a result of living in a stress-free environment such as the Dakota grasslands. Because the herds are smaller and the open pasture is cleaner than the feedlot, animals that graze on natural grasses do not depend on hormones or antibiotics. By allowing livestock to live in their natural environment, the meat is loaded with essential nutrients important for optimal health. Plus, it turns out that because grass-fed meats are higher in vitamin E, they actually stay fresher longer in stores and in your refrigerator.

The American Bison (Buffalo)

Imagine what Meriwether Lewis and William Clark witnessed as they trekked up the Missouri River and onto the open plains of the Dakotas during their famous cross-country expedition (1804–1806). It must have been an astonishing site for those early explorers, standing atop a hill and seeing tens of thousands of buffalo blanketing the landscape. At that time, the American bison (commonly known as the buffalo) numbered around 60 million and were free to roam most of the North American continent.

The buffalo was the center of life and part of the spiritual culture of the Plains Indians. Not only did the meat provide them with sustenance to survive, just about every part of the beast had a purpose or use. Its furry hide kept the tribe warm in the winter and its dung was used as fuel for fires. Buffalo bones were carved into needles and knives, and the horns made excellent cups and spoons. Even the tails were used for shooing flies.

This harmonious relationship between the Indian and the buffalo lasted for thousands of years. It took only a few decades of massive slaughter to leave the bison nearly extinct. The majority of the killings occurred between the 1830s and 1860s as wagon trains carted hides off to the east to be used in the production of clothing and belts. Leather and fur traders were not the only ones shooting the bison. United States government officials at the time promoted the destruction of the bison in order to control their Native American enemies. In 1876, Congressman James Throckmorton of Texas, feeling that it would help civilize the Indians, stated that it would be best if there was not "a buffalo in existence. Take away a nation's food supply and it is a lot easier to defeat them." Soon, the military was ordered to kill the buffalo in order to control the major food source of the Plains Indians. Hundreds of thousands of buffalo were arbitrarily slaughtered on a yearly basis, and by the end of the century, fewer than 1,000 remained.

In 1905, President Theodore Roosevelt convinced the U.S. Congress to establish a number of wildlife preserves for the buffalo. By 1929, almost 3,500 animals were counted. Ranchers soon began to realize the economic potential of the buffalo and were instrumental in rebuilding public and private buffalo herds. Today, the U.S. Department of Agriculture estimates that nearly 300,000 bison exist throughout the United States and North America.

The bison, once a symbol of strength and unity for the Plains Indians, we now know to be a nutrient-dense food. The proportion of protein, fat, minerals, and essential fatty acids in buffalo is high in relation to its caloric value. When compared to other animals from a feedlot, the bison have a greater concentration of iron and other essential nutrients. The meat from grass-fed bison can contain up to four times as much vitamin E as feedlot cattle. This potent antioxidant has been shown to lower the risk of heart disease, cancer, and Alzheimer's disease.

The fat content in bison meat is usually a third of that found in cattle fattened in the feedlot. Because the meat is lower in fat, it also means that it is lower in calories. A buffalo steak may have 100 fewer calories than a steak from a grain-fed steer. You could lose up to 10 pounds a year just by switching your main source of meat to grass-fed buffalo.

Bison meat is also high in omega-3 fatty acids. Omega-3s are formed in the chloroplasts of green leaves and as much as 60% of the fatty acid content in the grasses on the plains is omega-3; thus, buffalo allowed to graze on these natural grasses absorb these healthy fats. The benefits of a diet rich in omega-3 fatty acids cannot be overstated, ranging from cancer prevention to lowering cholesterol and reducing inflammation. Plus, because bison spend most of their lives eating grass, they are not subjected to drugs, hormones, or chemicals.

Bison meat has a similar flavor to fine beef, but I find it slightly sweeter and richer. Bison is a very lean red meat and it is best if not overcooked. Total cooking time will depend on the particular cut and thickness of the buffalo meat. Historically a key part of Native American culture, the popularity of the buffalo has returned to younger generations, who are beginning to restore this animal to the land. In a culture where obesity is in epidemic proportions, there couldn't be a better time for the buffalo to make a comeback.

"The buffalo meat, however, is the great staple and 'staff of life' in this country, and seldom (if ever) fails to afford them an abundant and wholesome means of subsistence. There is, from a fair computation, something like 250,000 Indians in these western regions, who live almost exclusively on the flesh of these animals, through every part of the year. During the summer and fall months, they use the meat fresh and cook it in a great variety of ways, by roasting, broiling, boiling, stewing, and smoking; and by boiling the ribs and joints with the marrow in them, make a delicious soup, which is universally used, and in vast quantities."

—GEORGE CATLIN, NORTH AMERICAN INDIANS

Lamb

When I was young, most families in America had only one television set with two stations to choose from, CBS or NBC. Since television was not the main source of entertainment, I found other ways to amuse myself. If I wasn't perfecting my abilities to tease or irritate my siblings, I was looking through the *World Book Encyclopedia* purchased by my mother, which covered nearly every subject from A to Z, and then some. As I was looking at the "S" book, I quickly turned to the section on South Dakota. I was proud to read that South Dakota is home to Mount Rushmore as well as the second largest gold mine in the world. My home state was also top in the nation's corn and wheat production, as well as the top sheep-producing state in the union. Sheep jokes aside, these were bragging rights for any nine-year-old who wanted to impress his cousins from another state.

Lamb meat was not a part of our diet. The only time we ate it was when my father ordered up a bunch of cubed mutton, skewered on a stick and fried in rendered sheep fat. He then would wash it down with a South Dakota Bloody Mary (tomato juice and beer). If you are dieting or trying to lower your cholesterol, this South Dakota treat is not for you.

Most Americans typically eat only a pound of lamb a year, as compared to 60 pounds of beef per year. In the past, sheep were bred primarily for wool and were not usually butchered until they served their purpose as wool producers. As a result, the meat was tough and had a gamey taste to it. Today, sheep are raised either for wool or for meat. Breeding methods have greatly improved the flavor and texture of lamb sold in this country.

TABLE 3.1. NUTRITIONAL PROFILE OF LAMB (Leg of lamb, roasted, 3 ounces)			
Calories	162	Cholesterol	75.7 mg
Total fat	6.58 g	Sodium	57.0 mg
Saturated fat	2.4 g	Riboflavin	0.2 mg
Monounsaturated fat	2.6 g	Niacin	6.0 mg
Polyunsaturated fat	0.46 g	Vitamin B_{12}	2.2 mcg
Protein	22.0 g	Phosphorus	165 mg
Carbohydrate	0 g	Zinc	3.9 mg

TABLE 3.2. LAMB VS. OTHER MEATS (PER 3-OUNCE SERVING)				
Meat	Calories	Fat	Saturated Fat	Cholesterol
Lamb leg (shank and sirloin)	162	6.58 g	2.4 g	75.7 mg
Pork (fresh ham)	179	8.02 g	2.8 g	80.2 mg
Beef round	164	6.59 g	2.4 g	69.0 mg
Chicken (dark and light)	162	6.32 g	1.7 g	75.3 mg
Turkey (dark and light)	145	4.23 g	1.4 g	64.4 mg

Lamb is an excellent source of protein, which the body uses to build and repair tissues. It is much leaner than beef, with a majority of its fat content in the form of either monounsaturated fats or omega-3 fats. It is also loaded with iron, which helps red blood cells carry oxygen to the body. Lamb is rich in a variety of B vitamins, such as niacin and B_{12}, which our cells need to function properly. Niacin also promotes healthy skin and nerves and has been proven to raise HDL (good) cholesterol and lower triglycerides in the body. Lamb also contains zinc, a mineral that the body needs for the production of enzymes and insulin. Zinc also helps to increase interferon levels in the lungs, helping to fight off viral infections such as the common cold.

Meat that is labeled "lamb" comes from yearling sheep, whereas mutton is sheep that is over two years old and is rarely sold as meat. A yearly mutton comes from a sheep that has been slaughtered between one and two years old. Lamb is naturally tender and does not need to be tenderized before cooking. Cooking times will vary with the size and cut of the meat. In general, the meat should be cooked slowly, over low to moderate heat, until the internal temperature is 135°F to 140°F. Braised or stewed lamb should be cooked to the desired degree of tenderness.

FISH OF THE DAKOTAS

Whether caught out of the vast oceans of the world or from the fresh lakes and streams of the Dakotas, fish and seafood are considered by most nutritionists a high-quality source of protein with fewer calories than red meat. Both fish and seafood contain B-complex vitamins that may help lower homocysteine levels in the blood. They are also rich in critical antioxidants such as vitamin E, which may prevent unstable oxygen molecules, or free radicals, from damaging LDL cholesterol, which is the first step in the buildup of coronary plaque. In addition to many other vitamins, including A and D, fish have several trace minerals, such as potassium, iron, phosphorus, copper, iodine, manganese, cobalt, and selenium.

Research regarding the health benefits of eating fish is ongoing, and much of the current investigation has focused on the kinds of fats in fish, particularly omega-3 fatty acids. Physicians and nutritionists are beginning to recommend more fish and seafood in the diet because of the health benefits of omega-3 oils and their effect on cholesterol and high blood pressure.

Although the fattier fish, such as salmon and trout, have more omega-3s than lean fish, even the leanest fish are good sources of this essential fat.

The number of calories per serving depends on the type of fish you consume and how it is prepared. For example, a 3-ounce filet of perch will have fewer calories then a 3-ounce Chinook salmon steak. Frying in oil will add more calories than broiling, poaching, or steaming. The use of condiments like butter or tartar sauce will also add a lot of calories. I recommend using fresh herbs such as curry powder, paprika, or sweet basil instead; a squeeze of lemon or lime juice can also enhance the flavor without raising the sodium content or adding calories.

Some sport fish caught in the Dakotas may contain elevated levels of mercury, which can pose a health risk if eaten in large amounts. The game, fish, and park departments of North and South Dakota have found that most of our lakes and streams have very low levels of mercury. But mercury is an issue in waters across the United States. If you are concerned about which bodies of water have mercury advisories, contact your local game, fish, and park departments for more information.

Chinook Salmon

Native to the Pacific Ocean and freshwater streams of the West Coast of North America, Chinook salmon were first introduced to the waters of the Missouri River back in the 1970s. They seem to do very well in the deep, cold reservoirs of lakes Sakakawea and Oahe and are stocked every spring in order to maintain the sport of fishing. Salmon are found in many parts of the United States and readily available in grocery stores everywhere. Salmon is rich in omega-3 fatty acids and low in saturated fat. It is also loaded with other vital nutrients and antioxidants that can improve your health.

When preparing salmon for cooking, never leave it at room temperature. If marinating, always do it in the refrigerator. Thaw frozen salmon overnight in the refrigerator as thawing at room temperature will allow bacteria to destroy its freshness. Salmon should be cooked thoroughly in order to destroy harmful organisms. The flesh should look opaque and flaky when done. Overcooking the fish will cause it to fall apart or become tough and dry. I recommend using a meat thermometer on large cuts of fish and taking the fish off the stove or grill when the core temperature reaches 145°F. Raw salmon in sushi bars or salmon prepared rare in restaurants is safe because the fish is frozen, which kills harmful parasites.

Trout

Brook, brown, and rainbow trout are very popular fish with anglers. Like salmon, trout is considered a fatty fish and is loaded with omega-3 fatty acids. Most species were introduced to the lakes and streams of the Dakotas and are typically stocked in the spring. Trout are usually found in many parts of the United States and also available in grocery stores. The flavor of trout is generally mild and sweet. The amount of omega-3 fats will vary depending on the size of the fish—generally, the larger the fish, the higher the fat content. Take the same precautions in preparing trout as you would with salmon. You can even substitute larger trout for salmon in many recipes.

Pike Family

There are two well-known species of pike that are native to the Dakotas, the northern pike and the muskellunge (or muskie). They are efficient predators that like cool clear waters as they use their keen vision to find their prey. Pike are one of the leanest of all fish, with less than 1 gram of fat per serving. The flesh is flaky dry, so I recommend either poaching or baking pike with a moist sauce.

Perch Family

The most well-known fish of this family are the walleye and yellow perch. Walleye are so called because of their large glassy pupil, which allows them to see well in low light conditions. Both types are native to North America and the Dakotas and are an excellent source of lean meat. Both are very healthy alternatives to red meat. Their flesh is flaky and white with a mild flavor, making them an excellent choice for the dinner table.

Bass and Sunfish Family

Bass and sunfish can be found in many of the lakes of the Dakotas and are extremely popular with anglers. Examples are both large and small mouth bass, crappie, and bluegill. They are fattier than the pike or perch family of fish, and therefore contain more omega-3s. They can be substituted in most fish recipes.

Catfish Family

The catfish is one of the most popular sport fishes and inhabits many waters of the Dakotas and in other parts of the United States. The fish has a smooth but tough skin that can be difficult to remove. They get their name from the four pairs of flexible barbels found on their head. This fish is very popular with American diners. It is low in calories and has a trace of omega-3 fatty acids.

We have now looked at some of the healthy foods included in the Dakota Diet—fresh fruits and vegetables, grains, nuts, meat, and fish. Incorporating more of these foods into you diet will provide a plethora of nutrients that can help you stay healthy and lose excess weight. Next, you'll find out how to start eating healthier according to the Dakota Diet plan.

CHAPTER 4

The Dakota Diet Plan

A re you ready to start your diet? When you are, remember to set realistic weight loss goals. Rapid weight loss will only lead to failure as you will most likely regain the weight you lost, and maybe even more. I recommend that you start slowly and make this the diet you will follow for the rest of your life. Does eating less mean that you have to give up all the things you used to enjoy? The answer lies in the quality of food you eat as well as the quantity. If you combine exercise with eating foods that are high in nutrients, then your meal portions do not have to change as drastically.

A HEALTHY BALANCE OF MACRONUTRIENTS

A commonsense approach to healthy eating is to balance the macronutrients—carbohydrates, fats, and protein. If weight loss is your goal, then reduce your total intake of calories each day and increase your expenditure of calories through exercise.

- Your total fat intake should be around 25% to 35% of daily calories, with less than 7% coming from saturated fat. The grass-fed animals of the Dakotas are nutrient-dense, low-calorie proteins, low in saturated fat, and high in omega-3 fatty acids.

- Total carbohydrates should range from 45% to 55% of your daily calories. Fiber is a carbohydrate and avoiding healthy carbs such as fiber can cause a multitude of problems, including constipation. Carbohydrates are a great source of energy and are important for a well-balanced diet.

65

- Protein intake should be between 20% and 25% of your daily calories. Protein comes from meat, eggs, dairy, and nuts. I recommend protein with every meal, as it will help reduce snacking between meals.

Getting a Healthy Balance of Fats

The Dakota Diet will give you a better balance of omega-6 to omega-3 fatty acids than the typical American diet consumed today. The grasses on the plains of the Dakotas have the nutrients to give us a healthy balance of fats. Buffalo, wild game, and cattle fed on the range are loaded with vital nutrients, iron, antioxidants, and a healthy ratio of omega-6s to omega-3s. When these animals are fed commercially (as in a feedlot), the ratio of omega-6s to omega-3s drastically changes for the worse. Range-fed animals of the Dakotas are not only lower in omega-6s and higher in omega-3s than their feedlot counterparts, they are also lower in unhealthy saturated fats and cholesterol.

Until the government and the food industry recognize the importance of eating a balanced ratio of essential fatty acids, you must learn to choose carefully. As you begin to read nutrition labels on the foods you shop for, look for the types of fats that will help safeguard your health. The Dakota Diet, which is based on the diet of the Mediterraneans, is free of artificial fats. What the Dakota Diet and the Mediterranean diet have in common is the foods consumed are free of trans-fatty acids (TFAs) and they are rich in omega-3 fatty acids. TFAs are artificial fats (hydrogenated and partially hydrogenated) that are detrimental to your health. It is important to choose cooking oils that are high in unsaturated fats and low in saturated ones (Table 4.1). By eating more fresh fruits and vegetables and foods rich in omega-3s (such as range-fed buffalo), your intake of TFAs is drastically reduced. You not only will lose the necessary weight, you will improve your cholesterol profile significantly without the need of expensive medications such as statin drugs. All it takes is a little knowledge and willpower in order to avoid the foods that are high in TFAs.

When you are grocery shopping, the first thing to do is spend some time reading product labels before you purchase the item. What you don't know about the foods you buy may in fact hurt you. By understanding what TFAs are and how they damage your blood vessels, you can choose foods free of hydrogenated vegetable oils and rich in omega-3 fats.

TABLE 4.1. DIETARY FATS: THE SATURATION SCALE		
Product	Saturated Fat (%)	Unsaturated Fat (%)
Canola oil	6	94
Safflower oil	10	90
Sunflower oil	11	89
Corn oil	13	87
Olive oil	14	86
Soybean oil	15	85
Margarine, tub	17	83
Peanut oil	18	82
Margarine, stick	20	80
Cottonseed oil	27	73
Solid vegetable shortening	32	68
Lard	41	59
Palm oil	52	48
Butter	66	34
Palm kernel oil	87	13
Coconut oil	92	8

Good Carbohydrates

Avoid simple carbohydrates such as white flour, sugars, and pastries. When wheat is refined and made into flour, the fiber is stripped away, making the carbohydrate or sugars in the flour much more easily absorbed in the digestive system. As a result, foods that are made of white flour, such as white bread, are simple carbohydrates that cause blood sugar to spike rapidly. When we eat a complex carbohydrate with the fiber preserved, this slows down the amount of carbohydrate or sugar absorbed, resulting in a lower blood sugar rise in the body.

Choose healthy carbohydrates such as multigrain breads, whole fruits, and vegetables. By eating carbohydrates that are slowly absorbed (complex carbohydrates), insulin is slowly released and the drop in blood sugar is less drastic. If you have better control of your blood sugar, then you will have fewer cravings for carbohydrates, which results in fewer calories consumed.

Finding Foods Free of Trans-Fat

Reading product labels may be time-consuming, especially if you have screaming kids demanding the latest and greatest breakfast cereal advertised on TV. The reward will come later as your children grow older, healthier, and wiser according to the types of foods they consume.

Fresh Fruits and Vegetables—All fresh fruits and vegetable are completely TFA free and are loaded with vitamins and other nutrients vital to your health. Preparing a meal from scratch may be difficult at times but can be a wonderful activity for the whole family to enjoy. If you are able to grow your own vegetables and fruits, you can enjoy the fruits of your labor all year long by freezing or canning what you have produced.

Meats, Fish, and Poultry—The diet of the Plains Indians included game that grazed on the native grasses or fish that survived in the clear lakes and streams of the Dakotas, providing a perfect, efficient, and healthy food source for these animals to survive in the wild. Unfortunately, the feedlot proved to be more profitable for the farmer, rancher, and big corporate agriculture. By feeding corn to cattle and poultry in a feedlot, the type of fat generated in their meat is drastically changed. TFAs are not present in any fresh meats; however, corn-fed meats and poultry are higher in saturated fats (known to raise LDL cholesterol) and omega-6 fats, with low amounts of omega-3 fats.

All fresh fish are free of TFAs. The fish of the Dakotas, such as Chinook salmon and brook and rainbow trout, are excellent sources of omega-3 fatty acids, unless they are from a fish farm. Just as cattle are raised to be fattened up in a feedlot, fish raised in this way will be lower in omega-3 fats and higher in saturated fat than those caught in the wild. The pike family of fish (walleye and northern) is also low in saturated fat and just plain great to eat if caught in a fresh lake. Some grocery stores may feature fresh fish and not farmed fish, and it is worth the trouble to seek them out.

Dairy Products—Essentially, dairy products are TFA free with the exception of imitation cheeses or canned milk products. It is import to read the label, and when choosing a product such as milk, try to reduce your total fat content by choosing 1% fat or skim milk. Cheese is an excellent source of protein with a low glycemic index; again, the lower the fat content, the better off you are.

Breads and Bakery Goods—Choose a multigrain or whole-grain bread rather than plain white bread, as the latter will cause your blood sugar to rise too fast. Some breads contain TFAs, so continue to be a conscientious label reader. Most bakery goods, such as pastries and doughnuts, are made with hydrogenated vegetable oils (TFAs), so you should keep the consumption of these items to a minimum or eliminate them altogether.

Cereals—Almost all boxed cereals contain TFAs in order to extend their shelf-life. Choosing cereals from a dry bin or natural food store is preferred as these products are usually free of TFAs.

Chips and Crackers—If you are attempting to lower your LDL (bad) cholesterol and trying to lose weight, I would recommend that you avoid all of these food items as they are loaded with TFAs. Not only will you get a hefty dose of trans-fats, but also the amount of carbohydrates will drive your pancreas wild.

Condiments—Read the labels when choosing salad dressings, ketchup, mayonnaise, and similar items. Most condiments are free of TFAs, and relishes and pickles are preserved in vinegar. If you are creative, you can always make fresh salsa or salad dressing from scratch.

Frozen and Snack Foods—Pizza, TV dinners, and frozen vegetables usually have sauces made from hydrogenated oils, so you will again have to be a label cop in order to purchase TFA-free products in the frozen food section. Breaded foods such as fish sticks, potato nuggets, and french fries have large amounts of TFAs and calories.

If you have to snack, choose foods that are high in fiber or complex carbohydrates. Snacking will not only provide additional calories, but the wrong snack will usually be loaded with TFAs. Candy bars, microwave popcorn, and chips and dips generally have high amounts of TFAs and calories.

If we only focus on a low-carbohydrate diet, we will be losing out on an excellent source of energy and other vital nutrients. Rather than eliminating or reducing carbohydrates, it is better to eat more complex carbohydrates that contain fiber, such as fruits and vegetables as well as whole multigrain breads. You should avoid simple carbohydrates such as white bread, pastries, and candy as their sugars are too readily accessible.

Recommended Grains

Barley	Oats
Buckwheat	Rye
Millet	Wheat

> Avoid simple carbohydrates such as white flour, sugars, and pastries. Choose healthy carbohydrates such as multigrain breads, whole fruits, and vegetables.

Fiber

Most Americans do not get enough fiber in their diet. The goal should be about 25 grams a day, but most of us get 10–15 grams a day. It is best if you start each day with a super-charged, fiber-rich breakfast, such as a bowl of your favorite bran cereal mixed with $\frac{1}{4}$ cup of ground flaxseed. Add two slices of toasted, stone-ground whole-wheat bread and you already have 17 grams of fiber for the day. (See Table 4.2.)

TABLE 4.2. SOURCES OF SOLUBLE FIBER		
Food	**Serving Size**	**Soluble Fiber per Serving**
Kidney beans	$\frac{1}{2}$ cup	3.0 g
Brussels sprouts	$\frac{1}{2}$ cup	3.0 g
Apple, with skin	1 medium	2.3 g
Pear, with skin	1 medium	2.0 g
Broccoli	$\frac{1}{2}$ cup	1.3 g
Carrot	1 large	1.3 g
Brown rice	$\frac{1}{2}$ cup	1.3 g
Oatmeal, cooked	$\frac{3}{4}$ cup	1.3 g
Orange	1 medium	1.3 g
Grapefruit	1 medium	1.3 g
Zucchini, cooked	$\frac{1}{2}$ cup	1.1 g
Barley	$\frac{1}{2}$ cup	1.0 g
Potato, baked with skin	1 medium	1.0 g
Strawberries	$\frac{3}{4}$ cup	0.9 g
Banana	1 medium	0.6 g

Fruits and Vegetables

I have often referred to the Dakota Diet as consisting of foods found right in our back yard. But this is not exclusive to the Dakotas—it includes any back yard that has the capability to support a vegetable garden. If you have the time and talent to undertake such a task, the rewards will be great. If not, then I would recommend seeking out your local co-op or farmer's market in to order get the freshest seasonal food available. Local supermarkets also offer a variety of fresh fruits and vegetables throughout the year.

We have known of the health benefits of fiber for years and are just beginning to realize the health benefits of consuming foods—particularly fruits and vegetables—rich in antioxidants and other phytonutrients (plant nutrients). Antioxidants include vitamins A, C, and E as well as trace minerals such as selenium and zinc. They work against the oxidative process, which causes cellular damage. Phytonutrients include the B vitamins, folic acid, flavonoids, and carotenoids. The best advice I can offer is to get your daily dose of antioxidants by eating five to eight servings of whole fruits and vegetables per day.

Recommended Fruits

Apples	Pears	Rhubarb
Blueberries	Plums	Strawberries
Cantaloupe	Raspberries	Watermelon

Recommended Vegetables

Asparagus	Cucumber	Parsley
Bell Peppers	Eggplant	Romaine Lettuce
Broccoli	Garlic	Spinach
Brussels Sprouts	Green Beans	Summer Squash
Cabbage	Green Peas	Tomato
Cauliflower	Kale	Turnip Greens
Celery	Leeks	Winter Squash
Collard Greens	Onions	

Recommended Root Vegetables

Beets	Horseradish	Yams
Carrots	Sweet Potatoes	

Recommended Legumes

Black Beans	Kidney Beans	Pinto Beans
Dried Peas	Lentils	Navy Beans

Protein

We need to retrain our thinking on what is produced and consumed in America. The common belief is that our palate finds marbled beef tastier, therefore the ranchers produce a meat with a higher fat content. When prepared properly, range-fed buffalo, game, and beef are just as palatable because they are grass-fed and have a blend of fats proven to promote optimal health. The meat from grass-fed animals has less fat and fewer calories than grain-fed animals. Additionally, the amount of omega-3 fat in the meat of grass-fed animals is higher, as is the amount of vitamin E and other nutrients. Bison (buffalo) is a healthy and delicious alternative to fattier beef and pork. Lamb is an excellent source of protein, which the body uses to build and repair tissues. It is much leaner than beef, with a majority of its fat content in the form of either monounsaturated fats or omega-3 fats. Fish and seafood are considered by most nutritionists a high-quality source of protein with fewer calories than red meat. Nuts and seeds are another excellent source of proteins as well as omega-3 fatty acids.

Recommended Proteins

American bison (buffalo)   Lamb   Wild game   Grass-fed beef

Fish—Chinook salmon, trout, pike family (northern pike and the muskellunge), perch family (walleye and yellow perch), bass and sunfish family (large and small mouth bass, crappie, and bluegill), catfish

Recommended Nuts

Flaxseed	Sunflower seeds	Pumpkin seeds
Walnuts	Almonds	

IMPLEMENTING THE DIET

Calorie counting can be difficult, especially if you are not preparing the food yourself. Calorie reduction, on the other hand, is more manageable and can be achieved even if you are mathematically challenged. If your weight has remained the same, despite increasing your activity, then you have to reduce your calorie intake for the day. In order to lose a pound a week, you must reduce your total calories by 600 calories a day.

Start a Food Diary and Exercise Journal

Being diligent in detailing what you eat will help you eliminate those foods that are high in calories and low in nutrients. Start a food diary, if you have not already done so. Keep a pencil and notebook handy and record what you eat throughout the day, and do this for at least a week. An ongoing food record will help you establish better eating habits and make you more accountable by discouraging mindless eating. Don't cheat—everything that goes into your mouth goes in your journal. Many of my patients tend to lose weight the first month after starting the diary as they avoid foods they would normally eat without thinking. The diary will make you account for the food that you eat, and often when the accountability factor is added, weight loss is achieved.

If you are keeping track of your daily caloric intake in order to manage your weight, you can easily count the calories in your diet by going to www.thecaloriecounter.com. Now, do the math. If you want to lose one pound a week, then you will have to eliminate at least 600 calories from your diet each day. One pound of fat equals approximately 455 grams, and there are 9 calories per gram of fat. Therefore, a pound of fat equals roughly 4,100 calories (that's equivalent to 19 Snickers bars). By reducing 600 calories a day, you will eliminate well over 4,100 calories and lose that pound in the first week.

The amount of calories you eat really depends on your age, sex, and whether you are an active or sedentary person (the latter is often the case for most people who are overweight). The key to dieting is eating foods that are healthier and low in calories. If you are not losing the weight you desire, then either reduce your portion size or increase your physical activity. If you diet without exercising, studies have shown that you can lose up to one pound of muscle for every three pounds of fat. Exercise will improve your lean body mass, and in turn will help you burn even more calories.

In addition to making you accountable for what you consume, a journal can also be useful for recording the type and amount of physical activity you perform each day. You can also keep track of your progress by charting your weight at least once a week, preferably at the same time of day. A weight chart can help you make the necessary corrections in your diet and exercise routine should you begin to gain some of the weight back.

Remove Temptations

Take an inventory of your home pantry. Replace your old cooking oil with canola or olive oil. Clean out your food pantry, throwing away all of the high-carbohydrate snack foods and other tempting foods that you know are bad for you. If you have to snack, eat walnuts, sunflower seeds, or almonds. They are not only filling but also loaded with nutrients and omega-3 fats, which can actually improve your cholesterol profile. Other nutritious snacks you can enjoy are sliced fruits and vegetables, which can be dipped in low-fat yogurt or fat-free ranch dressing. The spices found on your spice rack are okay, but fresh spices and herbs are even better. Fresh or frozen vegetables are better than canned vegetables, and whole-wheat pasta is better than white pasta.

Monitoring Your Progress

Step on the scale at least three times a week (preferably at the same time of day) and record your weight. By doing so, you will be monitoring your progress and can make adjustments to your diet and exercise as you see fit. When you reach your ideal body weight (see Tables 4.3 and 4.4), continue to weigh yourself to assure you that you keep the weight off.

THE DAKOTA DIET GUIDE TO SUCCESS

To begin your journey to healthier eating, remember the following guidelines:

- Eat at least five servings each of whole fruits and vegetables a day. By doing so, you will be certain to consume the necessary daily requirements

TABLE 4.3. IDEAL BODY WEIGHT BY HEIGHT AND FRAME—WOMEN

Height	Small Frame	Weight (in Pounds) Medium Frame	Large Frame
4' 10"	102–111	109–121	118–131
4' 11"	103–113	111–123	120–134
5' 0"	104–115	113–126	122–137
5' 1"	106–118	115–129	125–140
5' 2"	108–121	118–132	128–143
5' 3"	111–124	121–135	131–147
5' 4"	114–127	124–138	134–151
5' 5"	117–130	127–141	137–155
5' 6"	120–133	130–144	140–159
5' 7"	123–136	133–147	143–163
5' 8"	126–139	136–150	146–167
5' 9"	129–142	139–153	149–170
5' 10"	132–145	142–156	152–173
5' 11"	135–148	145–159	155–176
6' 0"	138–151	148–162	158–179

TABLE 4.4. IDEAL BODY WEIGHT BY HEIGHT AND FRAME—MEN

Height	Small Frame	Weight (in Pounds) Medium Frame	Large Frame
5' 2"	128–134	131–141	138–150
5' 3"	130–136	133–143	140–153
5' 4"	132–138	135–145	142–156
5' 5"	134–140	137–148	144–160
5' 6"	136–142	139–151	146–164
5' 7"	138–145	142–154	149–168
5' 8"	140–148	145–157	152–172
5' 9"	142–151	148–160	155–176
5' 10"	144–154	151–163	158–180
5' 11"	146–157	154–166	161–184
6' 0"	149–160	157–170	164–188
6' 1"	152–164	160–174	168–192
6' 2"	155–168	164–178	172–197
6' 3"	158–172	167–182	176–202
6' 4"	162–176	171–187	181–207

of vitamins and minerals. Whole fruits and vegetables are considered high-volume foods—high in fiber, water, and nutrients, and low in calories.

- Avoid processed foods and fast foods, as they are nutrient-poor and high in calories.

- Eat protein with every meal. This will help you feel full and prevent you from having hunger pangs two to three hours after a meal.

- Switch your regular consumption of fatty beef to leaner grass-fed buffalo. You could lose up to ten pounds the first year just by reducing the amount of fat calories in your diet.

- Avoid all foods containing trans-fatty acids, as they will destroy your cholesterol profile, raising your total and bad cholesterol and reducing your good cholesterol levels.

- Try to consume at least 30 grams of fiber per day, with at least 15–20 grams of fiber at breakfast.

- Drink a minimum of 64 ounces of water daily. Drink one glass before every meal, as this will aid in weight loss by filling you up faster. Dehydration can make you feel hungry. Drinking this amount of water will also help you avoid constipation, especially as you increase your intake of fresh fruits and vegetables.

- Eat often, at least five times a day, which will actually boost your metabolism and help you to burn more calories.

- Don't skip meals. This will lead to overeating and extra calories between meals that will be stored in the body rather than used as fuel for the day.

- Avoid eating foods high in carbohydrates right before bed. One of my patients had a bowl of breakfast cereal before he settled in for the night. By giving up this ritual, he was able to lose at least five pounds in a month without a major change in his lifestyle.

- Snack only on whole fruits, vegetables, and nuts.

- Exercise.

Breakfast

I recommend that you start your diet first thing in the morning. Research suggests that breakfast is the most important meal of the day. By eating breakfast, you will start your day having consumed most of your daily requirements of fiber, which will provide you with enough energy for the day and trigger your metabolism. You will find yourself eating fewer calories and snacking less by filling up on nutrient-dense foods of the Dakotas. By eating breakfast, you will not only have more energy, but you will also increase your metabolic (calorie burning) rate.

Avoid all refined sugars found in cereals and pastries. Whole-grain cereal is better, but don't be fooled by the general—General Mills, that is. Most processed cereals are loaded with simple sugars that add calories. Multigrain breads and fresh fruits are a much better choice.

Even if you are in a hurry, breakfast on the go should not consist of doughnuts or pastries. Your pantry should include healthy foods such as oatmeal, nuts, or even canned or dried fruit. Have a protein bar or fiber bar available for those "on the go" meals. Load up on fiber at breakfast: $\frac{1}{4}$ cup of ground flaxseed on bran cereal with two slices of multigrain toast provides up 17 grams of fiber.

Lunch

Your breakfast will get you through the morning and your appetite will be controlled by the water you drink throughout the day, and especially an hour or two before lunch. If you are at work and only are allowed half an hour for lunch, you might want to consider preparing your lunch at home. If time permits, then choose a restaurant offering healthy choices such as vegetable salads or soups. If you meet your friends or colleagues at the closest fast food restaurant, then your choice for healthy food will be limited. Plan ahead and don't pick a restaurant when you are hungry. Identify those that have healthy foods, make a list, and then choose your lunch spot from this list.

Drinking water, tea, or another diet drink will help you fill up without additional sugars from high-calorie beverages, including fruit drinks. Eat a protein, and if you desire something quick, always try to choose nature's fast food—whole fruits and vegetables.

Dinner

Preparing the evening meal is not only a great family activity but you also have control of the type and amount of food you will eat. Get your entire family involved in preparing the meal. This is a great way to spend quality time with your spouse and kids and educate them about food choices so they will incorporate these good eating habits into their lives. The amount of carbohydrates in this meal should be limited to less than 30% of your calories for the meal. Your breakfast and lunch should have given you the majority of this macronutrient for the day. Besides, you do not need a quick source of energy as the hour for sleep is just around the corner.

Snacks

If you have to snack, then choose nuts, whole fruits, or vegetables, or a protein such as cheese or yogurt. Avoid all simple carbohydrates, as this will only add unused calories and make you feel hungry again much sooner than healthier choices.

A 1,600-CALORIE MEAL PLAN FOR STARTERS

Below you will find a carefully designed 1,600-calorie daily meal plan that can serve as a guide to follow while dieting. If your hunger is not satisfied on this meal plan, then simply increase your portion size as you see fit. And remember, you are following this meal plan to not only help you lose weight, but also to help improve your overall health.

Day One

Breakfast

2 slices of multigrain bread with 4 tsp of natural peanut butter
Smoothie: 8 oz of skim milk, 2 tbsp of ground flaxseed,
$^1/_2$ cup of fruit (strawberries, blueberries, or other)

Lunch

Turkey sandwich: 2 slices of multigrain bread, 4 oz of sliced turkey breast,
lettuce, tomato, omega-3 (canola) butter for spread
8 oz of low-fat or skim milk
$^1/_2$ cup of baby carrots

Afternoon Snack

1 cup of fresh fruit or 6 oz of watermelon

Dinner

Buffalo Burger (see Appendix); you can substitute any lean meat
such as elk hamburger or grass-fed beef
Salad
3 ounces of grapes (10 grapes)

Evening Snack

6 cups of fat-free popcorn
Diet soda or water

DAILY TRACKER

Calories: 1,600	Cholesterol: 247 g
Total Fat: 52.9 g	Carbohydrates: 178 g
Saturated Fat: 11 g	Fiber: 17 g
Monounsaturated Fat: 16 g	Protein: 114 g
Polyunsaturated Fat: 14 g	Calcium: 875 mg
Omega-3s: 2.43 g	Sodium: 2.2 g

Day Two

Breakfast

1 cup of dry multigrain cereal with 6 oz of skim milk;
sprinkle with $\frac{1}{4}$ cup of ground flaxseed
1 cup of seasonal fruit

Lunch

Salmon sandwich: 2 slices of multigrain bread, 3 oz of fresh or
canned salmon, 2–5 pieces of watercress or other greens
1 cup sliced vegetables (your choice)
1 cup of fruit

Afternoon Snack

$\frac{1}{2}$ cup of low-fat cottage cheese, sprinkled
with 1 tbsp of ground flaxseed
$\frac{1}{2}$ cup of fruit

Dinner

Grilled Salmon Fillets, with Asparagus and Onions (see Appendix)
Salad greens with light dressing

Evening Snack

1 oz ($\frac{1}{4}$ cup) of nuts

DAILY TRACKER

Calories: 1,580   Cholesterol: 137 mg
Total Fat: 75 g   Carbohydrates: 150 g
Saturated Fat: 13   Fiber: 17 g
Monounsaturated Fat: 25 g   Protein: 98 g
Polyunsaturated Fat: 20.3 g Calcium: 837 mg
Omega-3s: 2.7 g   Sodium: 2 g

Day Three

Breakfast

1 slice of multigrain toast with 1 tsp of omega-3 butter
1 poached or hard-boiled omega-3 egg
$1/_2$ cantaloupe

Lunch

Chicken sandwich: 2 slices of multigrain bread, 2 oz of roasted (skinless) chicken, 1 oz low-fat or skim cheese, 1–2 slices of tomato, lettuce
1 cup of baby carrots
1 apple

Afternoon Snack

Light yogurt (90 calorie) sprinkled
with $1/_4$ cup of ground flaxseed

Dinner

Breast of Pheasant (Partridge or Quail) Cordon Bleu (see Appendix)
Tossed salad with low-calorie dressing
1 whole-wheat dinner roll

Evening Snack

3 oz of dried fruit

DAILY TRACKER

Calories: 1,615	Cholesterol: 424 mg
Total Fat: 75 g	Carbohydrates: 150 g
Saturated Fat: 24 g	Fiber: 17 g
Monounsaturated Fat: 20 g	Protein: 94 g
Polyunsaturated Fat: 15 g	Calcium: 600 mg
Omega-3s: 2.5 g	Sodium: 2 g

Shopping for the Right Foods

Here are a few practical tips for stocking up on healthier foods:

⊛ Buy only nutrient-dense, low-calorie foods as outlined in this book. A great source of protein is buffalo meat and other wild game or grass-fed cattle. Avoid all foods with trans-fatty acids, such as crackers and cookies. A good rule of thumb is that anything that has a long shelf life is likely not something you want to purchase or consume in large quantities.

⊛ Spend most of your time at the grocery store or local food cooperative in the fresh fruit and vegetable section. The local farmers market is a great place to find the freshest and best foods in your local area. The benefits of eating whole fruits and vegetables cannot be overstated.

⊛ Buy omega-3-enriched eggs. These are eggs produced by a hen allowed to graze free range. You can find them in most grocery stores, as their demand is on the rise. You may spend a bit more than for regular grade A eggs, but you are getting a great source of protein with the benefit of eating an egg enriched with omega-3 fats.

⊛ Have you "GOT MILK"? Then make it low in fat. If you grew up drinking whole milk, you may find it difficult to switch to skim overnight. I recommend that you slowly taper down to 2% milk, then to 1%, then skim.

⊛ Avoid all starchy foods, including white bread, white rice, and potatoes. The simple sugars in these foods are too easily absorbed, resulting in a spike of insulin.

Day Four

Breakfast

1 English muffin, toasted
1 slice of low-fat or skim cheese
Several tomato slices
1 cup of seasonal fruit

Lunch

Wild game wrap: 10-inch tortilla, 3 oz of skinless meat (your choice),
2 tbsp of salsa
2 cups of fresh fruit
1 cup of skim or fat-free soy milk

Afternoon Snack

1 cup of low-fat cottage cheese, sprinkled
with 1 tbsp of ground flaxseed
$^1/_2$ cup of fruit

Dinner

Prime Rib of Elk (see Appendix)
1 cup of yams or sweet potatoes
Salad greens with low-calorie dressing

Evening Snack

2 cups of fresh fruit

DAILY TRACKER

Calories: 1,600	Cholesterol: 188 mg
Total Fat: 43 g	Carbohydrates: 224 g
Saturated Fat: 14 g	Fiber: 21 g
Monounsaturated Fat: 10 g	Protein: 87 g
Polyunsaturated Fat: 9 g	Calcium: 893 mg
Omega-3s: 1.3 g	Sodium: 2.8 g

Day Five

Breakfast

1 cup of oatmeal sprinkled with 2 tbsp of ground flaxseed;
sweeten to taste with Splenda
$^1/_2$ cup of seasonal fruit

Lunch

Buffalo (or veggie) burger: 1 multigrain bun, 1 lean buffalo hamburger
or veggie patty, lettuce, tomato slice, mustard and/or catsup
Water or diet soda

Afternoon Snack

$^1/_2$ cup of walnuts

Dinner

Raspberry Salsa Walleye (see Appendix)
2 cups of steamed vegetables (your choice)
1 slice of Italian bread with 1 tsp of omega-3 butter

Evening Snack

4 wedges (approximately 1 cup)
of honeydew melon or watermelon

DAILY TRACKER

Calories: 1,612	Cholesterol: 293 mg
Total Fat: 81 g	Carbohydrates: 147 g
Saturated Fat: 13 g	Fiber: 21 g
Monounsaturated Fat: 25 g	Protein: 100 g
Polyunsaturated Fat: 37 g	Calcium: 625 mg
Omega-3s: 6.6 g	Sodium: 1.8 g

Day Six (The Weekend)

Breakfast

Dakota omelet: 2 omega-3 eggs, 1 tsp of canola oil,
1 oz of your favorite cheese, 1 tbsp of sun-dried tomatoes
1 cup of seasonal fruit or fat-free yogurt, sprinkled
with 2 tbsp of ground flaxseed
1 slice of multi-grain toast, with 1 tbsp omega-3 butter

Lunch

Chicken or wild game salad: 4 oz of skinless breast of wild game,
2 cups of greens, tomatoes, red pepper

Afternoon Snack

$3/_4$ cup of low-fat cottage cheese
$1/_2$ cup of fruit

Dinner

Angel Hair Pasta Mold (see Appendix)
Mixed salad

Evening Snack

$1/_2$ cup of apple sauce

DAILY TRACKER

Calories: 1,645   Cholesterol: 688 mg
Total Fat: 88 g   Carbohydrates: 113 g
Saturated Fat: 31 g   Fiber: 14 g
Monounsaturated Fat: 31 g   Protein: 100 g
Polyunsaturated Fat: 15 g   Calcium: 770 mg
Omega-3s: 2.6 g   Sodium: 3.0 g

Day Seven (Fun Day on Sunday)

Breakfast

2 buttermilk or whole-grain pancakes (pre-mixed),
with 2 tbsp of ground flax meal added;
1 tsp of omega-3 butter, 2 tbsp of light maple syrup
$^1/_2$ cup of sliced fruit

Lunch

Salad: 2 cups of greens, $^2/_3$ cup of garbanzo beans, $^3/_4$ cup of broccoli
or other vegetable, 2 tbsp of low-calorie salad dressing
1 small whole-wheat roll
Skim milk or fat-free soy milk
$^1/_2$ cup of sliced fruit

Afternoon Snack

12 ounces of tomato or V-8 juice
$^1/_4$ cup of nuts

Dinner

Romantic Dinner for Two with Lamb Chops (see Appendix)
Heart Soup (see Appendix)

Evening Snack

$^2/_3$ cup of low-fat cottage cheese

DAILY TRACKER

Calories: 1,680	Cholesterol: 211 mg
Total Fat: 69 gm	Carbohydrates: 113 g
Saturated Fat: 18 g	Fiber: 31 g
Monounsaturated Fat: 15 g	Protein: 79 g
Polyunsaturated Fat: 23 g	Calcium: 890 mg
Omega-3s: 2.5 g	Sodium: 4 g

How Sweet It Is

The next time you reach for the sugar bowl to sweeten your favorite cereal or fruit, try an artificial sweetener instead. All sugars such as powdered, granulated, or brown sugar, fructose (found in fruits), lactose (milk), and maltose (beer) contain calories. By substituting an artificial sweetener, you can reduce the overall calories and help manage your weight.

Sugar used in baking goods not only adds sweetness to the product, it also caramelizes as it cooks and helps yeast breads to rise. Many of the newer substitutes can be used in place of sugar as they are heat stable and acceptable for baking. Add them at the end of the recipe to maximize the sweetening effect.

Honey is another alternative that can be used in place of sugar in most recipes. Honey is sweeter than sugar, so you will want to use less ($\frac{1}{2}$ to $\frac{3}{4}$ cup for each cup of sugar). Honey not only has fewer calories than sugar, it also provides antioxidants such as vitamin B_2, vitamin B_6, iron, and manganese.

The following are some of the most common sugar substitutes:

Saccharin—Products such as Sweet 'n Low, Sugar Twin, and Weight Watchers Sweetener contain this artificial sweetener. Saccharin can be used in baking goods and is up to 380 times as sweet as traditional table sugar.

Aspartame—This sugar substitute, better known as NutraSweet or Equal, was approved by the U.S. Food and Drug Administration (FDA) in 1974 and can still be found in a number of products, such as soft drinks, puddings, and frozen desserts. I would not use this in baking as the molecule is altered in the heating process.

Ascesulfame K—The FDA approved the use of ascesulfame K in 1987 and it is now found in chewing gums and dessert mixes and is used as a table sugar known as Sweet One.

Sucralose—This product was approved in 1998 and is better known as Splenda. It is a sugar substitute made directly from the sugar molecule and is extremely heat stable. My wife and I use it to sweeten bitter things such as fruit for our kids. I especially like it because it does not have an aftertaste like many other artificial sweeteners on the market.

Using artificial sweeteners as a substitute for sugars will not only help you control your calories, they also do not promote tooth decay and are not considered harmful to humans at the levels normally used. The sugar alcohols (sorbitol, lactilol, mannitol, maltitol) used to sweeten "sugar-free" candy or gum have fewer calories than sugar and do not cause a sudden increase in blood glucose because they are not easily absorbed by the body. In excess, however, sugar alcohols can have a laxative effect.

Prior to 2000, foods and beverages that contained saccharin had warning labels because of findings that it caused bladder tumors in mice when given in high doses. Recent studies have not shown an increase in the risk of these types of cancer, prompting the U.S. Congress to pass legislation removing the warning label. Additionally, the National Cancer Institute claims no scientific evidence that any of the artificial sweeteners cause cancer and they are considered safe for use by the general population.

People with a rare metabolic hereditary disease known as phenylketonuria (PKU) should avoid all products that contain aspartame as the artificial sweetener is synthesized from aspartic acid and phenylalanine, two essential amino acids. Aspartame has also been linked to migraine headaches. People with sensitivity to the food flavor enhancer monosodium glutamate (MSG) may also react if they ingest foods or beverages containing aspartame.

Remember, just because you reduce the amount of calories in your cooking by substituting artificial sweeteners for sugar, if you eat too much, you will still be getting more calories than you need. Choosing sugar-free soft drinks, desserts, or candy are considered empty calories and will provide no important nutrients, unlike the foods of the Dakota Diet.

Day Eight

Breakfast

Toasted bagel with 1.5 oz of lox (cold smoked salmon),
sun-dried tomatoes, capers
1 slice of melon (water or honeydew)

Lunch

Turkey sandwich: 2 slices of multigrain bread, 4 oz of sliced turkey breast,
lettuce, tomato, omega-3 (canola) butter for spread
8 oz of low-fat or skim milk
$^1/_2$ cup of baby carrots

Afternoon Snack

$^1/_2$ cup of seasonal fruit

Dinner

Lake Trout Baked with Herbs (5 oz) (see Appendix);
you can substitute any fish such as salmon or walleye
Salad: Baby greens with dried pine nuts and diet Italian dressing

Evening Snack

6 cups of fat-free popcorn
Diet soda or water

DAILY TRACKER

Calories: 1,652	Cholesterol: 221 g
Total Fat: 62 g	Carbohydrates: 158 g
Saturated Fat: 15 g	Fiber: 22 g
Monounsaturated Fat: 20.7 g	Protein: 107 g
Polyunsaturated Fat: 20 g	Calcium: 613 mg
Omega-3s: 1.2 g	Sodium: 2.5 g

Day Nine

Breakfast

1 cup of dry multigrain cereal, with 6 oz of skim milk;
sprinkle with 2 tbsp of ground flaxseed
1 cup of seasonal fruit

Lunch

Turkey sandwich: 2 slices of multigrain bread, 4 oz of sliced turkey breast,
lettuce, tomato, omega-3 (canola) butter for spread
8 oz of low-fat or skim milk
$^1/_2$ cup of baby carrots

Afternoon Snack

1 cup of fresh fruit

Dinner

Deer/Venison Chili (see Appendix); you can substitute any lean meat
such as elk, buffalo, or grass-fed beef
2 small whole-wheat rolls
Skim milk or fat-free soy milk

Evening Snack

Diet soda or water

DAILY TRACKER

Calories: 1,611	Cholesterol: 246 mg
Total Fat: 42 g	Carbohydrates: 202 g
Saturated Fat: 10 g	Fiber: 20 g
Monounsaturated Fat: 10 g	Protein: 920 g
Polyunsaturated Fat: 17 g	Calcium: 919 mg
Omega-3s: 5 g	Sodium: 3.5 g

Day Ten

Breakfast

1 cup of non-fat yogurt, sprinkled with 1 tbsp of ground flaxseed;
add 1 cup of seasonal fruit

Lunch

Salmon sandwich: 2 slices of multigrain bread, 3 oz of fresh or canned
salmon, 2–5 pieces of watercress or other greens
$^1/_2$ cup sliced vegetables (your choice)
1 cup of fruit

Afternoon Snack

1 cup of low-fat cottage cheese, sprinkled with
1 tbsp of ground flaxseed
$^1/_2$ cup of fruit

Dinner

Parmesan Turkey Breast (see Appendix)
Salad greens with light dressing

Evening Snack

$^1/_2$ cup of seasonal fruit

DAILY TRACKER

Calories: 1,645	Cholesterol: 143 mg
Total Fat: 55 g	Carbohydrates: 171 g
Saturated Fat: 21 g	Fiber: 26 g
Monounsaturated Fat: 14 g	Protein: 104 g
Polyunsaturated Fat: 15 g	Calcium: 1,000 mg
Omega-3s: 3.12 g	Sodium: 3.2 g

Day Eleven

Breakfast

1 slice of multigrain toast with 2 tsp of jam
1 poached or boiled omega-3 egg
$^1/_2$ cup of seasonal fruit

Lunch

Salmon sandwich: 2 slices of multigrain bread, 3 oz of fresh or canned
salmon, 2–5 pieces of watercress or other greens
$^1/_2$ cup of sliced vegetables (your choice)
1 cup of fruit

Afternoon Snack

1 cup of low-fat cottage cheese, sprinkled
with 1 tbsp of ground flaxseed
$^1/_2$ cup of fruit

Dinner

Bison Kabob (see Appendix)
Barley Salad with Shallot Vinaigrette (see Appendix)

Evening Snack

2 oz ($^1/_2$ cup) of nuts

DAILY TRACKER

Calories: 1,650   Cholesterol: 244 mg
Total Fat: 53 g   Carbohydrates: 200 g
Saturated Fat: 11 g   Fiber: 34 g
Monounsaturated Fat: 20 g   Protein: 103 g
Polyunsaturated Fat: 13 g   Calcium: 570 mg
Omega-3s: 1.73 g   Sodium: 2 g

Day Twelve

Breakfast

1 English muffin, toasted
1 slice of low-fat or skim cheese
Several tomato slices
1 cup of seasonal fruit

Lunch

Salmon sandwich: 2 slices of multigrain bread, 3 oz of fresh or canned
salmon, 2–5 pieces of watercress or other greens
$^1/_2$ cup of sliced vegetables (your choice)
1 cup of fruit

Afternoon Snack

1 cup of low-fat cottage cheese, sprinkled with 1 tbsp of ground flaxseed
$^1/_2$ cup of fruit

Dinner

Breast of Pheasant (Chicken, Partridge, or Quail) Cordon Bleu (see Appendix)
Salad: mixed baby greens with diet salad dressing or vinaigrette
$^1/_2$ cup of seasonal fruit

Evening Snack

2 oz ($^1/_2$ cup) of nuts

DAILY TRACKER

Calories: 1,603	Cholesterol: 236 mg
Total Fat: 60 g	Carbohydrates: 186 g
Saturated Fat: 22 g	Fiber: 16.6 g
Monounsaturated Fat: 18 g	Protein: 80 g
Polyunsaturated Fat: 15 g	Calcium: 850 mg
Omega-3s: 1 g	Sodium: 3 g

Day Thirteen (The Weekend)

Breakfast

Vegetable omelet: 1 cup of fresh vegetables,
1 omega-3 egg plus two egg whites
1 slice of multigrain toast with 1 tsp of omega-3 butter

Lunch

Salmon sandwich: 2 slices of multigrain bread, 3 oz of fresh or
canned salmon, 2–5 pieces of watercress or other greens
$^1/_2$ cup of sliced vegetables (your choice)
1 cup of fruit

Afternoon Snack

$^1/_2$ cup of fruit

Dinner

Grilled Buffalo (or Beef) Ribs (see Appendix)
Salad: Baby greens with diet salad dressing
$^1/_2$ cup of seasonal fruit

Evening Snack

$^1/_2$ cup of seasonal fruit

DAILY TRACKER

Calories: 1,668	Cholesterol: 333 mg
Total Fat: 51 g	Carbohydrates: 155 g
Saturated Fat: 16 g	Fiber: 14 g
Monounsaturated Fat: 20 g	Protein: 134 g
Polyunsaturated Fat: 12 g	Calcium: 603 mg
Omega-3s: 0.82 g	Sodium: 2.2 g

Day Fourteen (Fun Day)

Breakfast

Two 5-inch Blueberry Flax Pancakes (see Appendix),
with 2 tbsp of pure maple syrup
6 oz of skim milk

Lunch

Wild game wrap: 10-inch tortilla, 4 oz wild game
(chicken, turkey), 1 cup of vegetables
of your choice, $\frac{1}{4}$ cup of salsa
2 cups of fruit

Afternoon Snack

1 cup of low-fat cottage cheese
$\frac{1}{2}$ cup of fruit

Dinner

Mediterranean Lamb Stew (see Appendix)
Curried Red Lentil Soup (see Appendix)

Evening Snack

2 tbsp sunflower seeds

DAILY TRACKER

Calories: 1,636	Cholesterol: 260 mg
Total Fat: 55 g	Carbohydrates: 190 g
Saturated Fat: 17 g	Fiber: 15 g
Monounsaturated Fat: 17 g	Protein: 98 g
Polyunsaturated Fat: 14 g	Calcium: 913 mg
Omega-3s: 1 g	Sodium: 2.5 g

HEALTHY COOKING TIPS

When you are trying to lose weight or lower your cholesterol, how you prepare your food is just as important as what you eat. Never fry foods, as this
only adds unnecessary calories and fat to your meal. If you have heart failure
and have to avoid salt or sodium, you do not have to give up the foods you
love. A few minor changes in preparing your meal will go a long way toward a
healthier diet.

- Poach chicken or fish by simmering it in a hot liquid. You can heat it to the
  temperature you want without the added fat of frying.

- The microwave works well for many foods as a fast alternative to frying.

- Grilling or broiling meats in the oven will allow the fats to drip away.

- When baking foods, use covered cookware with a little extra liquid.

- Steam vegetables over simmering water; that way, the vegetables will
  retain more of their flavor and nutrients.

- Use a wok to stir-fry vegetables and meat with vegetable stock, wine, or a
  small amount of canola or olive oil.

- Roasting meats prevents the food from sitting in its own fat drippings. Use
  fat-free liquids such as wine or lemon juice instead of the pan drippings
  when basting. Gravy can be made from the drippings by using a strainer or
  skim ladle to remove the fat.

- When sautéing, use a nonstick pan, as it allows you to use little or no oil as
  you cook.

    You can make your favorite recipes healthier by substituting or cutting
down on the content of fat without sacrificing the flavor.

- If your recipe calls for whole milk, use skim milk instead, and add one
  tablespoon of unsaturated cooking oil or canola oil.

- Use low-fat cottage cheese and nonfat yogurt if your recipe calls for sour
  cream (fat-free sour cream is also available).

- Evaporated skim milk works well instead of heavy cream.

- If your recipe calls for butter, use a polyunsaturated spread like Smart Balance or an omega-3 spread.

- One egg white plus 2 teaspoons of canola oil will work equally as well as one whole egg. Omega-3-enriched eggs are the healthiest option.

TIPS FOR EATING AT RESTAURANTS

Just because you're on a diet does not mean that you have to give up the things you enjoy. Life would be exhausting if you had to prepare all of your meals at home. In many American families, both parents work outside the home, and the children are involved in a number of extracurricular activities. My wife and I are both working physicians, with three children, including twins in the stage of life known as the "terrible twos." The task of preparing a meal at home after a busy day can be overwhelming, and the clean-up can be just as daunting. It is no wonder that many Americans spend up to 40% of the time eating out at restaurants or fast food joints.

The boredom of dieting can be a huge obstacle to overcome, but eating out at restaurants can be just as challenging. Restaurants generally serve two to three times the recommended amount of calories per serving. As soon as you sit down, your server brings an endless pile of chips or plate of bread, and then you're offered appetizers and a salad. The main entrée is then served, followed by dessert. Wash all of this down with a couple of alcoholic drinks and you have exceeded your total calories for the day. As a result of public demand, more and more restaurants are now offering healthier choices. Owners of restaurants, however, want to satisfy their customers as well as their hunger. The pitfalls of dieting and eating out are not what you eat but—equally important—how much you eat. Preparing a meal at home is usually a better idea, if you have the time. Even though restaurants are offering healthier choices, you still have to limit the amount of food you eat:

- Have 1–2 glasses of water at least an hour before your meal. This will help you feel less hungry by the time your food is served.

- Avoid the endless pit of free chips, bread, or crackers that are typically offered before the meal is served. Instead, ask for a salad right away, with the dressing on the side for dipping, or order a vegetable plate as a healthy appetizer.

- Consider ordering a la carte, such as salad and soup with an appetizer.

- Share a meal with dining partners. Most restaurants provide you with enough food and are usually willing to accommodate this request.

- Watch the fat. Avoid or limit the cream-based sauces. You can be assured that anything fried is not a good choice, so make substitutions by asking for fresh fruit or vegetables.

- Limit alcohol consumption. A couple of beers or glasses of wine can add as much as 300 calories to your meal. Quench your thirst right away with either a glass of water or iced tea.

- If you are on the road, avoid stretches of four or five hours between meals. The goal is to avoid feeling hungry and then overeating at a restaurant. You'll end up overindulging on the foods that are served and feel guilty about failing your diet.

- Don't be a plate cleaner. Many of us will clean our plates regardless of our appetite. Ask for a takeout box for the leftovers and enjoy them for lunch the next day.

- Always choose a low-calorie salad before your main entrée, as this will satisfy your hunger. Waiting awhile (up to 20 minutes) after eating the salad before consuming the rest of your meal will give your body time to adjust and often results in a greater sense of fullness.

- Make sure that your meal includes a source of protein, such as meat, fish, or poultry. Vegetarians can choose a dairy product. This will help prevent you from feeling hungry within a few hours after you have eaten.

CHAPTER 5

Get Fit and
Stay Slim

Health results from a harmony between food and exercise.
–HIPPOCRATES

It seems that the predominant subject on the news lately is the growing problem of obesity. Obesity refers to people who are overweight, often with a multitude of health problems related to their obesity, including heart disease and diabetes. Obesity is the number one most preventable cause of disease in our society. I think that physicians should write an "exercise prescription" for all of their patients with high cholesterol, as it has been shown to protect the heart by raising good cholesterol and lowering bad cholesterol levels. It also improves blood flow to all of the cells in the body (including the heart), providing them with proper nutrients and antioxidants to keep them healthy and prevent disease. Blood glucose is utilized more efficiently, thus helping to lower your risk of developing diabetes and even controlling blood sugar in diabetic patients.

It might be better to use the phrase "caloric imbalance" to describe the 60% of Americans who are considered overweight. Simply put, it is a matter of too many calories coming in and not enough calories going out. A calorie is a unit of heat equal to the amount required to raise 1 gram of water 1 degree Celsius. Calorie control is one of the most important methods of controlling your weight and improving your health.

But exercise is also part of a healthy lifestyle and a major component in the Dakota Diet plan. Maintaining an active lifestyle will help you lose weight and keep it off for good. The U.S. Surgeon General recommends at least 30 to 60 minutes of vigorous activity a day. If you are like many Americans, finding the time to exercise may be difficult. Keep in mind, however, that all types of physical activity add up in a day. For example, brief bouts of physical activity—such as taking the stairs instead of the elevator or walking for 10 minutes after breakfast, lunch, and dinner—will eventually get you to your goal. Exercise can come in many other forms and can be as simple as vacuuming, raking leaves, and washing the car.

You can fundamentally change your life by incorporating work activities and household chores into your exercise routine. Even lifting the laundry basket full of clothes 20 times before doing the laundry will tone your muscles and burn calories. Chopping wood, mowing the lawn, and gardening will spruce up your property as well as your body. For example, a 140-pound person doing the following household chores for twenty minutes will burn up a surprising number of calories:

Activity	Calories Burned	Activity	Calories Burned
Dusting	75	Scrubbing floors	175
Gardening	150	Shoveling snow	190
House cleaning	110	Stacking firewood	195
Ironing	70	Sweeping	80
Making the bed	70	Vacuuming	80
Mowing the lawn	150	Washing the car	140
Painting home	160	Washing the dishes	70
Moving furniture	210	Washing windows	145

FOR THE BEGINNER

If you lead a sedentary life and want to become more physically active, the activity should be started slowly and gradually increased in small increments. By slowly increasing your training, your muscles and ligaments will begin to move more freely, making you less likely to sustain an injury.

Walking is one of the easiest activities to help you achieve your goal. Not only is it cheap to perform, but you can also do it just about anywhere. It is also considered a weight-bearing activity, which means that it will improve muscle mass and help to strengthen the bones. Start by walking for at least

30 minutes a day. A pedometer (available at sporting goods stores) can calculate how many steps you take (2,000 steps equals one mile) and even determine the amount of calories you burn during your walk. Depending on your weight, whether you walk or run, the amount of calories you burn in one mile is fairly constant. A 140-pound person will burn up to 80 calories a mile, whereas a 200-pound person will burn up to 110 calories walking the same distance. Essentially, the more "baggage" you carry, the more calories you burn. You can easily calculate how many calories you will burn per mile just by starting with 80 calories, then adding 5 calories for every 10 pounds over 140 pounds you weigh. Or start with 80 calories, then subtract 5 calories for every 10 pounds under 140 pounds you weigh.

With time, depending on the amount of weight lost, you may start to engage in more strenuous activities such as cycling, cross-country skiing, and jogging. Your health-care provider will be able to evaluate your ability to perform such activities. Always get a check-up before engaging in more strenuous activities. Age alone should not prevent you from activity. If you are over 65 years old and overweight, a weight-loss program should consist of proper nutritional and exercise counseling in order to address important aspects of nutrition and minimize the likelihood of injury when you start to exercise.

If you prefer working out at the gym, then I would seek out a fitness trainer, who can assess your physical condition and start you on a program that is suited to your needs. Having a trainer with regular appointments will serve as a motivation for you to succeed. Many people feel intimidated in the gym or don't have time to go to a gym. A fitness trainer can work with you in order to create an exercise routine to fit into your busy lifestyle.

The bottom line with starting an exercise program is reducing the amount of sedentary time spent watching television or working on the computer. As you start to increase your activity level, not only will you start to burn the calories you consume, but you will also benefit your body in many other ways. For example, your lean body mass will improve (less fat and more muscle). As a result, you will burn even more calories, because muscles require more energy.

My philosophy for weight loss has always been "slim slow"—the same is true for physical activity. Start slow, gradually increasing the activity. Trying too hard at first can lead to failure and even injury.

Getting Started

Get into a routine of walking, starting out slowly and building up to 30 to 40 minutes each day. Remember, it all adds up, so you can get this amount of exercise by walking to work or taking the stairs instead of the elevator. Try walking after breakfast, lunch, and dinner. This is a great way to get started on a routine that will have tremendous health benefits. Once this becomes routine, then you can advance your pace and intensity level for a good cardio-vascular workout.

When you are able to comfortably walk for 15 to 20 minutes, increase your pace or the duration of a walk just enough so that you can hold a conversation with your walking partner without getting winded. Try to keep your heart rate at 75% of your maximum predicted heart rate (maximum heart rate equals 220 minus your age).

As you start to pick up your pace and effort, include a warm up before and cool down after your walk. Your warm up should include a stretching period to increase your flexibility and help prevent injury. It is good to stretch after your exercise as well, because the muscles are now warmed up and more pliable. Think of your muscles as being like saltwater taffy—when the taffy is cold, it won't stretch much, but let the taffy sit in the sun and it will stretch nicely. Warm up your muscles with exercise and then stretch them. Spend one-third of the total stretching time before exercise and two-thirds of your total stretching time after exercise.

If you want the extra challenge and want to burn off even more calories, then simply add periods of higher intensity (at least three minutes) to your walking routine. An example of this would be to add running up a hill or the stairs at home for a brief period of time, followed by an easy walk. What you are trying to do is to increase your heart rate to at least 85% of your maximum. It is important to remember to properly warm up and stretch in order to avoid injury to the joints and muscles in the body and only increase the intensity once you have mastered the 20 minute walk with your heart rate in the target zone of 65%–75% of maximum.

Adding these bursts of very high intensity activity can have a very positive effect on your weight loss and conditioning. A recent study suggests that bursts of very high intensity can result in significant increases in the release of growth hormone, which will help promote weight loss and increase lean muscle mass. As your conditioning improves, start a program where you sprint for up to 30 seconds and then walk for 90 seconds. Do eight cycles of this program to maximize your exercise program.

Get your upper body involved in the work out by pumping your arms as you walk. By doing so, you can increase the number of calories burned by as much as 10%. If you have a treadmill, try to avoid resting your arms on the handle in front of you as this will, for obvious reasons, reduce your calorie burn.

Walking is a great way to get started on a healthy lifestyle. As your body begins to demand more oxygen for fuel while exercising, the supply line (the arteries delivering the oxygen) will improve as well. These are the nuts and bolts of aerobic activity, which will improve your health as well as help you lose weight and keep it off forever.

Start Strength Training

Your exercise program will not be complete until you add strengthening exercises to your routine. What you are attempting to do is build and tone muscles in the body. You might want to find a trainer to help figure out how much weight to start with in order for you to maximize your weight training workout without injuring yourself. A trainer can also design a program that is unique to your abilities and lifestyle. If you decide to do this on your own, here are some guidelines that you should follow as you start.

- Do at least two sets of 10 repetitions with the weight you choose. If you cannot complete the workout, then you are using too much weight. If it is too easy, add more weight rather than more repetitions with the same weight.

- Exhale as you lift or contract the muscles and inhale as you relax.

- Give each muscle group a day of rest. In other words, work the upper body one day and the lower body the next day.

- Emphasize good technique. Sloppy lifting doesn't effectively isolate the muscle and will result in slower improvement of individual muscle groups.

- Develop a program that you can do at home so that if the weather is bad you don't have an excuse to not work out.

- Start with a program that focuses on core strengthening (strengthening of the abdominal muscles).

A strengthening program will benefit you as you build lean muscle and eliminate more fat. Muscles require more energy, thus boosting your metabolism. It also will help you to build stronger bones.

NUTRITION, PHYSICAL EDUCATION, AND "NO CHILD LEFT WITH A BIG BEHIND"

Intelligence and skill can only function at peak
when the body is healthy and strong.
—PRESIDENT JOHN F. KENNEDY

As a physician, I have to admit that most of my training on nutrition was limited to several brief lectures during the first two years of medical school. Yet, one of the first orders of business I perform when a patient is admitted to the hospital is determining what kind of diet they should follow. The diets to choose from are generally well thought out and tailored to the type of patient being admitted. Simply put, people with high blood pressure or those with heart failure are put on a salt-restricted diet, whereas those with coronary artery disease usually follow a low-cholesterol, low-fat diet. All diabetic patients get a carbohydrate-restricted diet, and those with morbid obesity will get their calories restricted. Further instructions as to what type of diet to follow at home will commence prior to being dismissed from the hospital.

Unfortunately, most physicians don't have time to discuss a diet plan with their patients during office visits. We spend most of our time treating the disease rather than preventing what got the person into trouble in the first place.

Even though our nutritional education was limited in medical school, I can sum up what I learned in one sentence: The more you eat, the fatter you become. Who needs to spend any more time on the subject than that? As the old saying goes, "you are what you eat." No lecture on nutrition is going to teach me that. I see it first-hand on a daily basis. A fast food nation is what we demand, and the food industry has responded with quick, fatty, unhealthy foods. As a result, we are the fattest nation in the world. Now that we are suffering from obesity, our society now wants a "slim fast" plan to correct the problem. Rather then focusing our limited medical resources on prevention of obesity, we spend billions of dollars treating diseases related to obesity, such as diabetes and heart disease. One thing is for certain, we will bankrupt our children's future if we continue this trend.

We cannot leave it up to the medical schools to teach future physicians the basics of nutrition—we must start a lot earlier than that. Our public and private schools must find a way to change the way our children think about food. More than 9 million children and adolescents between the ages of 6 and 19 are considered overweight. According to the U.S. Centers for Disease Control (CDC), if a child between the ages of 6 and 12 is overweight, the probability of that same child being overweight as an adult is roughly 50%; for adolescents, the probability increases to nearly 80%. As obesity increases in our youth, so will the diseases of the future.

Children at risk who do not eat right will end up suffering from diabetes and heart disease as a result. Just like overweight adults, obese children are more commonly diagnosed with high blood pressure, sleep apnea, liver disease, and diabetes. Obese children often experience low self-esteem and depression, which can lead to other poor choices, such as smoking and alcohol consumption.

With nearly two-thirds of our adult population considered to be overweight, some would imply that the problem with childhood obesity is genetic. I would argue that, in most situations, overeating is more a learned behavior than some sort of vicious gene passed on from parents. Consuming too many calories with minimal physical activity is mainly why we have an obesity epidemic in this country.

Not only should more be done in nutritional education at the elementary level, our school lunch menu needs to change as well. In the last two decades, children have begun to consume a greater number of calories each day and their choices in food have a higher fat content. The school systems should offer a healthier lunch menu rather than allowing the student an opportunity to purchase their foods or beverages from a vending machine. Parents have to play a major role in this as well. Mothers and fathers need to

Body Mass Index (BMI)
for Adults and Children

Body mass index (BMI) is a formula used to identify obesity as well as the degree of total body fat. These measurements help to identify who is at risk for high blood pressure, diabetes, and other diseases associated with obesity. The BMI is a measurement of a person's weight in kilograms divided by the square of their height in meters. It can also be calculated by dividing your weight in pounds by the square of the height in inches, then multiplying the result by 703.

Adults with a BMI between 18 and 25 are considered normal. If the BMI falls between 25 and 30, then you are considered overweight. A person is considered obese if their BMI is greater than 30.

Children differ from adults in that their body fat varies more as they grow. A child's BMI is plotted on a growth curve that reflects the age and sex of the child. Percentile scores are then used to determine whether a child is overweight, underweight, or obese. The U.S. Centers for Disease Control has BMI growth charts available online at http://www.cdc.gov/growthcharts. If a child's BMI-for-age is 5% or below, then they are considered underweight. Children with a BMI-for-age between 6% and 85% are generally considered to be at a healthy weight. A BMI-for-age between 85% and 95% place that child at risk for becoming overweight, and anything above 95% is considered to be overweight.

If you are concerned that your child is overweight, I recommend that you seek medical advice from a qualified physician to evaluate the child for other disorders, such as high blood pressure and high cholesterol. Since children are still growing, weight loss is not usually recommended. It is best to try to maintain the child's baseline weight, as this will result in a gradual reduction in BMI as the child grows. Weight loss is usually recommended if a child between the ages of 2 and 7 has high blood pressure, high cholesterol, or other complications. For children older than 7 years, weight loss is recommended if the BMI-for-age is greater than 95% or if it is between 85% and 95% with high cholesterol, high blood pressure, or other complications.

be just as concerned about what their children are eating in school as they are about what they are learning in school. In order to reverse the obesity trend, we need to start early in life by educating and encouraging healthy food choices. I would encourage all parents to get involved by changing the way we think about nutrition. The health and welfare of our children is our future. Once the public demands change, our food industry and government bodies will follow suit in order to make that change happen. Our government needs to address childhood obesity now or suffer the long-term financial consequences of treating complications of obesity. Perhaps they can call their new initiative "No Child Left with a Big Behind."

Active Kids are Healthy Kids

Like many American adults, children do not follow a healthy eating plan or get involved in physical activity for a variety of reasons. Leaving a child at home with the TV, computer, or video games for entertainment only encourages our children to be sedentary. As parents, we should find other activities for our children after school. An organized recreational school program like tennis or soccer is a great example.

Recently, my mother visited us, and my 8-year-old daughter, Josie, attempted to get her grandma to play with her. Grandma told her that she would play with her after she was done exercising. Josie then reminded us all that playing is exercising. Having family activities such as playing tag, going on a nature hike, or playing an organized sport is a great way for the whole family to keep in shape.

Unfortunately, many public schools are giving up recess in order to meet the mandates set forth by the government in No Child Left Behind. Students at risk for falling behind have to forgo physical education and recess in exchange for additional study time. According to the National Association for Sports and Physical Education, the majority of high schools in the United States require students to take only one year of physical education in order to graduate. But the U.S. Surgeon General recommends that children engage in moderate physical activity for at least 60 minutes a day.

Parents and educators must take an active role in addressing childhood obesity. We must not only give our children a chance to make the right nutritional choices, we have to lead by example. I doubt patients would take my medical advice to lose weight and quit smoking if I were an obese smoker myself. The same is true for parents and educators. We may teach nutrition and physical education in health class, yet schools sometimes contradict those messages with the choices that are offered in the lunch room and hallway vending machines. Recess is taken away from students and physical education is no longer a priority. This lethal combination has resulted in an epidemic of obesity in our youth.

ACTIVITIES TO BURN CALORIES

"A flaw in the human character is that everybody wants to build and nobody wants to do maintenance."

–KURT VONNEGUT

You can get your exercise and burn off calories and pounds just by living your life! Below you will find a list of activities, ranging from common household chores to occupations to sports, and how many calories they burn. Depending on your weight, the amount of activity and calories burned will vary, as will the time spent doing the activity. Multiply the number of calories you burn per minute by the number of minutes you perform the activity. You'll probably be surprised to see how many calories you consume in your normal daily activities. Source: American College of Sports Medicine. "Compendium of Physical Activities: An Update of Activity Codes and MET Intensities." *Medicine & Science in Sports & Exercise* (September 2000).

CALORIES BURNED PER MINUTE FOR DIFFERENT BODY WEIGHTS						
	100 lbs	120 lbs	140 lbs	160 lbs	180 lbs	200 lbs
Activity in a Physical Fitness Center or Gym						
Aerobics, low-impact	5	6	7	8	9	10
Aerobics, high-impact	7	8	10	11	13	14
Aerobics, step	9	10	12	14	15	17
Aerobics, water	4	5	6	6	7	8
Bicycling, stationary (moderate)	7	8	10	11	13	14
Bicycling, stationary (vigorous)	11	13	15	17	19	21

	100 lbs	120 lbs	140 lbs	160 lbs	180 lbs	200 lbs
Calisthenics, vigorous (jumping jacks, push-ups, sit-ups)	8	10	11	13	14	16
Circuit training	8	10	11	13	14	16
Elliptical trainer	7	9	10	12	13	14
Rowing, stationary (moderate)	7	8	10	11	13	14
Rowing, stationary (vigorous)	9	10	12	14	15	17
Ski machine	7	8	10	11	13	14
Stair-step machine	9	11	13	14	16	18
Stretching	3	3	4	4	5	5
Weight lifting, light (free weights, nautilus, or universal)	3	3	4	5	5	6
Weight lifting, vigorous (free weights, nautilus, or universal)	6	7	8	10	11	12
Sports Activity or Training						
Archery	4	4	5	6	6	7
Badminton	5	5	6	7	8	9
Basketball	8	10	11	13	14	16
Billiards	3	3	4	4	5	5
Bicycling, BMX or mountain	9	10	12	14	15	17
Bicycling, 12–13.9 mph, moderate effort	8	10	11	12	14	16
Bowling	3	4	4	5	5	6
Boxing, sparring	9	11	13	14	16	18
Boxing, punching bag	6	7	8	10	11	12
Coaching (football, soccer, basketball)	4	5	6	6	7	8
Dancing, fast (disco, ballet)	5	6	6	8	9	9
Dancing, slow (waltz, foxtrot)	3	4	4	5	5	6
Fencing	6	7	8	10	11	12
Football, competitive	9	11	13	14	16	18
Football, touch or flag	8	10	11	13	14	16

	100 lbs	120 lbs	140 lbs	160 lbs	180 lbs	200 lbs
Football, playing catch	3	3	4	4	5	5
Frisbee, ultimate	8	10	11	13	14	16
Golf, carrying clubs	5	5	6	7	8	9
Golf, using cart	4	4	5	6	6	7
Gymnastics	4	5	6	6	7	8
Hacky-sack	4	5	6	6	7	8
Handball	12	14	17	19	22	24
Hiking	6	7	8	10	11	12
Hockey, field or ice	8	10	11	13	14	16
Horseback riding	4	5	6	6	7	8
Ice skating	7	8	10	11	13	14
Kayaking	5	6	7	8	9	10
Martial arts (judo, karate, kickboxing, Tae Kwan Do)	10	12	14	16	18	20
Motor-cross	4	5	6	6	7	8
Polo	10	12	14	16	18	20
Racquetball	10	12	14	16	18	20
Rock climbing	11	13	15	18	20	22
Rope jumping	10	12	14	16	18	20
Running, 5 mph (12 min/mile)	8	10	11	13	14	16
Running, 6 mph (10 min/mile)	10	12	14	16	18	20
Running, 7 mph (8.5 min/mile)	12	14	16	18	21	23
Scuba diving	7	8	10	11	13	14
Skateboarding	5	6	7	8	9	10
Skiing, cross-country (light)	7	8	10	11	13	14
Skiing, cross-country (vigorous)	9	11	13	14	16	18
Skiing, downhill (light)	6	7	8	10	11	12
Skiing, downhill (vigorous)	8	10	11	13	14	16
Snow shoeing	8	10	11	13	14	16

	100 lbs	120 lbs	140 lbs	160 lbs	180 lbs	200 lbs
Soccer	10	12	14	16	18	20
Softball or baseball, slow or fast pitch	5	6	7	8	9	10
Squash	12	15	17	19	22	24
Surfing, body or board	3	4	4	5	5	6
Swimming, leisurely	6	7	8	10	11	12
Swimming, laps	10	12	14	16	18	20
Table tennis or ping pong	4	5	6	6	7	8
Tai Chi	4	5	6	6	7	8
Tennis, singles	8	10	11	13	14	16
Tennis, doubles	5	6	7	8	9	10
Track & field: shot, discus, hammer throw	4	5	6	6	7	8
Track & field: high jump, long jump, triple jump, javelin, pole vault	6	7	8	10	11	12
Track & field: steeplechase, hurdles	10	12	14	16	18	20
Volleyball, non-competitive	3	4	4	5	5	6
Volleyball, competitive	8	10	11	13	14	16
Walk, 2 mph (30 min/mile)	3	3	4	4	5	5
Walk, 3 mph (20 min/mile)	3	4	5	5	6	7
Walk, 4 mph (15 min/mile)	5	6	7	8	9	10
Walk, 5 mph (12 min/mile)	8	10	11	13	14	16
Water skiing	6	7	8	10	11	12
Water polo	10	12	14	16	18	20
Water volleyball	3	4	4	5	5	6
Home Repair and Improvements (Outdoors)						
Carpentry, installing rain gutters, building fences	6	7	8	10	11	12
Carrying and stacking wood	5	6	7	8	9	10

	100 lbs	120 lbs	140 lbs	160 lbs	180 lbs	200 lbs
Chopping and splitting wood	6	7	8	10	11	12
Cleaning rain gutters	5	6	7	8	9	10
Digging, spading dirt, composting	5	6	7	8	9	10
Gardening	4	5	7	6	7	8
Laying sod/crushed rock	5	6	7	8	9	10
Mowing lawn, push, hand mower	6	7	8	10	11	12
Mowing lawn, push, power mower	6	7	8	9	10	11
Operating snow blower, walking	4	5	6	7	8	9
Paint outside of home	5	6	7	8	9	10
Planting seedlings, shrubs, trees	5	5	6	7	8	9
Raking lawn	4	5	6	7	8	9
Roofing	6	7	8	10	11	12
Sacking grass or leaves	4	5	6	6	7	8
Shoveling snow	6	7	8	10	11	12
Storm windows, hanging	5	6	7	8	9	10
Sweeping sidewalks	4	5	6	6	7	8
Trimming shrubs/trees, manual cutter	5	5	6	7	8	9
Trimming using edger, power cutter, etc.	4	4	5	6	6	7
Watering/fertilizing plants	3	3	4	4	5	5
Workshop, general carpentry	3	4	4	5	5	6
Home Repair and Improvements (Indoors)						
Carpentry, finish or refinish furniture	5	5	6	7	8	9
Caulking, bathroom, windows	5	5	6	7	8	9
Hang sheet rock, paper or plaster walls	3	3	4	5	5	6

	100 lbs	120 lbs	140 lbs	160 lbs	180 lbs	200 lbs
Lay or remove carpet/tile	5	5	6	7	8	9
Paint, paper, remodel	5	5	6	7	8	9
Sanding floors with a power sander	5	5	6	7	8	9
Wiring and plumbing	3	4	4	5	5	6
Activities in the Office						
Driving vehicle to work	2	2	3	3	4	4
Riding in a bus or vehicle to work	1	1	1	2	2	2
Sitting, light office work, meetings	2	2	2	2	3	3
Standing, filing, light work	2	2	3	4	4	5
Typing (computer, electric, or manual)	2	2	2	2	3	3
Walking during work break	4	4	5	6	6	7
Occupational Activities						
Bakery	4	5	6	6	7	8
Bartending/server	2	2	3	3	4	4
Building road, hauling debris, driving heavy machinery	6	7	8	10	11	12
Carpentry work	4	4	5	6	6	7
Coaching sports	4	5	6	6	7	8
Computer work	2	2	2	2	3	3
Construction, remodeling	6	7	8	9	10	11
Custodial work	4	4	5	6	6	7
Electrical work	4	4	5	6	6	7
Firefighting	12	14	17	19	22	24
Forestry, planting trees by hand	6	7	8	10	11	12
Heavy equipment operator	3	3	4	4	5	5
Horse grooming	6	7	8	10	11	12

	100 lbs	120 lbs	140 lbs	160 lbs	180 lbs	200 lbs
Locksmith	4	4	5	6	6	7
Masonry	7	8	10	11	13	14
Masseur	4	5	6	6	7	8
Patient care, nursing	3	4	4	5	5	6
Plumbing	4	4	5	6	6	7
Shoe repair	3	3	4	4	5	5
Steel mill	8	10	11	13	14	16
Truck driving, loading and unloading truck	7	8	9	10	12	13
Welding	3	4	4	5	5	6
Activities of Daily Living						
Child-care (bathing, feeding)	3	4	4	5	5	6
Cleaning house	3	4	4	5	5	6
Cooking/food preparation	2	2	3	3	4	4
Food shopping, with or without cart	2	3	3	4	4	5
Heavy cleaning (washing car or windows)	3	4	4	5	5	6
Ironing	2	3	3	4	4	5
Making bed	2	2	3	3	4	4
Moving household furniture	6	7	8	10	11	12
Playing with kids	4	5	6	6	7	8
Reading	1	1	1	2	2	2
Sleeping	1	1	1	1	2	2
Vacuuming	4	4	5	6	6	7
Watching TV	1	1	1	2	2	2

CHAPTER 6

The Dakota Diet
and Disease Prevention

We have to give a lot of credit to our mothers for constantly reminding us to eat our fruits and vegetables. Nutritional and health research has finally supported mom's claim that eating fresh fruits and vegetables will make us healthy and strong. Even the new food pyramid from the U.S. Department of Agriculture (USDA) supports this claim. But despite everything learned over the last several decades on obesity and disease, research into nutrition and health still lacks funding. Research efforts are focused on the treatment of diseases rather than prevention. At the same time, health-care costs in the United States are predicted to rise dramatically as the population ages. According to the U.S. government, one in every $5 will be spent on health care by 2015 and annual health-care spending will exceed $4 trillion. Common sense dictates that we implement a more preventive strategy, emphasizing healthier eating and exercise. What we now know is that eating whole fruits and vegetables and the right fats—as in the Dakota Diet—can reduce your risk of developing a number of diseases, including heart disease and cancer.

HEART DISEASE

Labor Day in 1981 was the day my father passed away. He was only 55 years old, playing volleyball with his seven children while his only grandchild watched from the sideline. He fell to his knees, with a clenched fist to his chest, and passed away despite every effort to revive him. We could only assume that my father's sudden death was a result of a heart attack due to underlying heart disease. I was only 19 years old at the time, yet it was evident to me that my father had many of the risk factors for heart disease, such as smoking and a high-stress job. Little did I realize that his sedentary lifestyle and high-calorie diet would lead to central obesity, which alone is a major risk factor for diabetes and heart disease. It was decades of exposure to this type of lifestyle that led my father to his premature death.

In the years since then, we have gained a better understanding of the causes of strokes and heart attacks. As a result of expensive interventions such as heart catheterizations and bypass surgery, we have seen a decline in the death rate from heart disease. Yet, despite this wealth of knowledge, we still spend over $300 billion a year treating heart disease rather then preventing it from happening in the first place.

More than 600,000 deaths occur each year from heart disease; 1.5 million Americans will suffer a heart attack this year, and one-third of those people will not survive the event. The more risk factors you have, the greater the chances of suffering a heart attack, so take the necessary steps to reduce your risk of heart disease. You may prolong your life, but more importantly, improve your quality of life. Had my father changed some things in his life, he would be playing volleyball with his family today, and enjoying the quality of life many of his peers enjoy. Instead of one grandchild sitting on the sideline watching him play volleyball, there would be 17 grandchildren playing with him, admiring his youth and agility.

Heart Disease Risk Factors

Most physicians spend a great deal of time and effort educating patients on ways to modify those risk factors that lead to heart disease and strokes. Many patients take expensive medications in order to treat their high blood pressure or high cholesterol. The price of these drugs can be high, but so is their effectiveness. Newer and safer medications are constantly being developed. Taking these medications in order to lower blood pressure or blood cholesterol has been shown to reduce the risk of heart disease, strokes, and diabetes. The research into lifestyle changes is just as powerful. By exercising, eating the right amounts of fats, such as those fats outlined in the

Dakota Diet, and avoiding carbohydrates that are easily absorbed, you may be able to significantly reduce the chance of developing heart disease.

There are unfortunately other risk factors for heart disease that cannot be changed but can be managed, such as the aging process and a family history of heart disease. The following is a list of risk factors and ways to slow down the disease process.

Changeable Factors

Smoking—Smoking raises your heart rate and blood pressure, making more work for your heart. Plus, blood clots more easily and arteries constrict. Your heart muscle is more likely to have rhythm irregularities. There is evidence that nicotine (the chief addictive component of tobacco) directly affects the arteries by damaging the lining, accelerating arteriosclerosis. Quitting smoking will have an immediate benefit on your heart and lungs, not to mention your pocketbook.

High Blood Pressure—You are at higher risk for heart disease if your blood pressure is greater than 135/90. Higher pressure means more work for your heart and damage to the lining of arteries, leading to a heart attack or stroke. If you are prescribed blood pressure medications, continue to take them, lose weight, reduce your salt and alcohol intake, and get regular exercise.

High Cholesterol—A total cholesterol greater than 200 and HDL (good) cholesterol of less than 45 places you at a higher risk for heart disease. Higher cholesterol in the blood causes a faster build-up of plaque in the arteries. Your target should be a total cholesterol of less than 200, triglycerides of less than 150, HDL (high-density lipoprotein) greater than 45, and an LDL (low-density lipoprotein or bad cholesterol) of less then 100. You can lower your total cholesterol by following the dietary guidelines of the Dakota Diet, as well as lower your LDL and raise your HDL.

Excess Weight—More weight means more work for your heart and may lead to high blood pressure and diabetes. Reducing your total calorie intake and increasing your daily activity level, as with the Dakota Diet, may help you avoid these problems.

Stress—Negative thoughts and responses to stressful situations burden the heart with more work and make it susceptible to life-threatening rhythm irregularities.

Lack of Activity—An inactive lifestyle at home or work increases your risk of heart disease. Begin and maintain a program of regular aerobic exercise. Walk more, use the stairs, and park your car in the farthest space in the lot and walk. You will be amazed at the health benefits of an active lifestyle and you may reduce your risk of a heart attack by as much as 50%.

Unchangeable Factors

Age—Your risk for heart disease increases as you get older.

Gender—Men are at greater risk for heart disease than women. This risk, however, is equal when women reach menopause.

Diabetes—Uncontrolled diabetes greatly increases heart disease risk. Weight loss and exercise can increase your body's ability to use insulin and glucose, causing some forms of adult-onset diabetes to disappear.

Family History—If one of your first-degree relatives had their first heart attack before the age of 55, you are at increased risk for heart disease. It is imperative that you attempt to reduce the number of risk factors, such as quit smoking, lose weight, exercise, control your blood pressure, and control your blood sugars if you are a diabetic.

High Cholesterol

Did you know that the human body has over 60,000 miles of blood vessels? This network is like a river delivering nutrients and oxygen to our cells. When this blood vessel river flows freely, it efficiently transports its life-sustaining cargo, which helps keep our bodies healthy. If the river becomes blocked, illness and disease can occur because our cells do not receive an adequate supply of nutrients and oxygen. As we age, our blood vessels may become blocked. The blockage is often the result of hardening and narrowing of the arteries caused by plaques that build up in our arteries.

The main culprit causing this build-up of plaques is cholesterol. Though it can cause problems in our blood vessels, cholesterol is vital to our bodies. Cholesterol is used to make hormones and vitamins, is part of our cell walls, and is involved in producing bile acids, which help the body process fats.

How does a substance vital to our health also cause such problems? When there is too much cholesterol in our bodies, the excess can build up in the walls of our arteries, causing them to harden (arteriosclerosis). As the arteries narrow, the heart may get less oxygen, which weakens the heart muscle and chest pain (angina) will occur when the heart is stressed. If a blood clot forms in the narrow artery, a heart attack (myocardial infarction) or even death can result.

More than 100 million American adults have elevated blood cholesterol levels, which is one of the key risk factors of heart disease. Therefore, it is important to understand what cholesterol is and how it affects your health. The buildup of cholesterol in the arteries is a slow process. By lowering high blood cholesterol, you can slow down this process or even reverse the buildup, thus lowering your risk for heart disease.

Cholesterol is a fat derived from both animal and vegetable sources. When doctors measure cholesterol, they look at total cholesterol and also measure lipoproteins, high-density lipoproteins (HDLs) and low-density lipoproteins (LDLs). Just like oil and water, cholesterol and blood do not mix. In order to travel in the bloodstream, cholesterol is coated with a layer of protein, making a lipoprotein. LDLs carry most of the cholesterol to the cells and are the main source of dangerous buildup and blockage in the arteries: the more LDL in the blood, the greater the risk of heart disease. HDLs carry excess cholesterol that is not used by the cell and deliver it to the liver to be removed from the body. HDLs help to keep cholesterol from building up in the walls of the arteries. If your level of good cholesterol (HDLs) is low, your risk of heart disease is greater.

There are many factors that determine whether your blood-cholesterol level is high or low. Your genes might determine the amount of cholesterol your body makes, as high blood cholesterol can run in families. A diet high in saturated fats (found mostly in foods that come from animals) and trans-fatty acids (found in margarines and other processed foods) can raise your cholesterol level more than anything else. An important first step in lowering your cholesterol is to follow a diet such as the Dakota Diet, which is low in these types of bad fats.

If you are overweight and lead a sedentary lifestyle, you may have a tendency for high cholesterol. Losing weight, as well as regular physical activity, may help lower your LDL cholesterol and raise HDL cholesterol levels. The proper amount of exercise can help you burn off more calories and improve your cholesterol profile.

Women tend to have lower cholesterol then men of the same age. As a woman gets older and reaches menopause, there is an increase in LDL cholesterol levels. Some women may benefit from taking estrogen after menopause, as it will lower LDLs and raise HDLs.

Manage Your Cholesterol with Diet and Exercise

Whether you have heart disease or want to prevent it, you can reduce your risk of heart disease by lowering your cholesterol level. Along with exercise, the Dakota Diet will not only help you achieve you ideal body weight, but also provide you with a rich supply of antioxidants, monounsaturated fatty acids, and omega-3 fatty acids. It will also provide you with a safe level of saturated fat and omega-6 fatty acids. The Dakota Diet will provide you with the necessary ingredients for a healthy heart.

As our society has become more overweight, the number of Americans with high cholesterol has increased as well. How much cholesterol you have in your body is greatly influenced by the types of food that you eat. In the past, most physicians would prescribe a diet low in cholesterol and fat as the first line of defense against high cholesterol. We now know that this was not such a good idea. As our society started to consume more foods claiming to be low in fat, we started to gain weight and worsen our cholesterol profile. In order to make the low-fat product taste better, the food industry added simple carbohydrates such as fructose and other sugars. By replacing the fat in the product with sugars, they added a lot of unnecessary calories.

It is possible to manage your cholesterol with diet alone. The Dakota Diet focuses on replacing harmful fats with healthier fats and eating more fruits and vegetables, rather than eating simple carbohydrates and foods loaded with trans-fatty acids as seen in many processed and convenience foods. No more than 35% of daily calories should come from fat and no more than 7% of the fat should be saturated fat. Saturated fat and trans-fatty acids are found primarily in animal products and hydrogenated vegetable oils and are major contributors to high cholesterol levels. Polyunsaturated fats, such as omega-3 fatty acids, and monounsaturated oils are healthier and should be used in place of saturated oils such as coconut oil, shortening, and lard.

As we age, our cholesterol profile changes as a result of increased body fat, which causes LDL to rise. Additionally, HDL levels drop due to unpredictable hormone levels, poor diet, and lack of physical activity. If you have high cholesterol and you are told to go on a low-fat diet and do not reduce your calories, your cholesterol will not change all that much. The body processes fats in the diet by breaking them down into a substance known as acetone, which in turn is used to make cholesterol. When you restrict your calories, the body uses the acetone for energy rather than diverting it to the liver for the production of cholesterol.

If you have high cholesterol, your doctor will prescribe a program of diet, exercise, and weight loss in order to bring levels down. You should try this for at least a six-months before considering drug therapy. Don't get too discouraged if you see only a small rise in HDL levels—even a small increase can help protect your arteries from developing plaque. Sometimes diet and exercise alone are not enough to lower your cholesterol. In these cases, your doctor may prescribe cholesterol-lowering medications.

Whether you have heart disease or want to prevent it, you can reduce your risk for having a heart attack or a stroke by lowering your blood cholesterol. Following a diet consisting of foods on the Dakota Diet will help you lower your total cholesterol and shed a few pounds in the process.

Foods and Nutrients

There are a number of individual foods that may help lower blood cholesterol without the use of medications. By making a few changes in the types of food you eat, you may be able to slow down or even reverse the build-up of fatty deposits in the walls of arteries. The following is a list of nutrients and foods proven effective in lowering blood cholesterol. Some are not necessarily found on the plains of the Dakotas but are nutritionally important and should be included.

Chromium—Foods such as nuts, oysters, and mushrooms contain large amounts of chromium. It may help lower LDL cholesterol and raise HDL cholesterol levels, as it appears chromium helps break down fats in the diet.

Copper—There is some evidence that a diet low in copper is linked to high levels of LDL cholesterol and a decrease in HDL cholesterol. Foods such as mushrooms and shellfish are leading food sources of copper.

Soluble Fiber—Carrots, beans, barley, oats, and apples are high in soluble fiber. They contain beta-glucan, a substance that interferes with the absorption and production of cholesterol.

Flavonoids—Researchers believe that foods high in flavonoids may block the production of LDL cholesterol and raise HDL levels. Foods such as broccoli, blueberries, tomatoes, apples, limes, onions and grapefruit are loaded with flavonoids.

Garlic—Garlic contains allinin and allicin, which are believed to interfere with the metabolism of cholesterol in the liver. They may also lower the amount of cholesterol released into the bloodstream.

Lycopene—Researchers believe that lycopene may interfere with the body's ability to make cholesterol by inhibiting an enzyme (HMG-CoA reductase) in the liver used to produce cholesterol. Tomatoes, grapefruit, and watermelon contain lycopene.

Omega-3 Fatty Acids—The Dakota Diet features this essential fatty acid. Numerous studies have demonstrated a link between a reduction in heart disease risk and a higher intake of omega-3s. People who consume salmon, trout, range-fed buffalo, and flaxseed have shown a significant drop in LDL cholesterol levels.

Polyphenolic Compounds—These are very potent antioxidants that may prevent the formation of LDL cholesterol. They can be found in alcoholic beverages such as wine.

Pantothenic Acid—Also known as vitamin B_5, pantothenic acid appears to lower the amount of fats in the blood. It can be found in foods such as avocado, salmon, sunflower seeds, yogurt, and mushrooms.

Soy Isoflavones—Soybeans, tofu, and other soy products contain isoflavones, which may help to lower LDL and total cholesterol while boosting the heart-protective HDL cholesterol.

Vitamin E—Vitamin E (alpha-tocopherol) seems to prevent unstable oxygen molecules (free radicals) from damaging LDL cholesterol, which is the first step in the build-up of coronary plaque. A recent study found that there was an increased risk of death (by 5%) when people took more then 400 international units (IU) of vitamin E daily. Vitamin E appears safe at low doses and may prevent Alzheimer's disease and boost your immune system. Most of us get up to 200 IU in our diet from nuts, seeds, and green leafy vegetables as well as grass-fed meats.

Vitamin C—This well-known vitamin may help to protect the bad cholesterol (LDL) from oxidation, thus preventing plaque build-up in the coronary arteries. Vitamin C also enhances the effect of vitamin E in the fight against high cholesterol.

Exercise

Research has shown that combining a calorie-reduced diet with regular physical activity can significantly improve cholesterol levels. Exercise works its magic by raising the good cholesterol (HDL) and lowering bad cholesterol (LDL). Even a single episode of physical activity can result in an improved cholesterol profile that persists for several days.

There are multiple reasons for high levels of cholesterol in the blood; certainly, genetics plays a major role for many Americans. Even with a proper diet and exercise, the cholesterol profile may not change all that much in those who are genetically predisposed to high cholesterol. Exercise still can play a major role in the prevention of death due to heart disease. A study published in the *Journal of the American Medical Association* found that men could reduce their risk of death from heart disease by 37% and women could reduce their risk by around 48% if they exercised on a regular basis. Another study published in *Circulation* found that men can cut their risk of dying from heart disease in half by being physically fit, regardless of their cholesterol level.

If you decide to begin an exercise program, understand your limitations and seek advice from your doctor before doing anything too vigorous. Multiple studies have shown that even increasing your everyday activities, such as walking the dog an additional 10 minutes or taking the stairs instead of the elevator, can have a positive impact on your health. Any type of activity can offset the problems associated with a sedentary lifestyle. (See Chapter 5 for more tips on beginning an exercise program.)

Testimonial: The Dakota Diet Lowers Cholesterol

"I have to admit that I never thought that what I ate really mattered much," says Jeff. "In my early adult years, I felt healthy, full of energy, and was free of disease. Then came the monumental age of 40 and my yearly physical with Dr. Weiland. To my surprise, my cholesterol was out of control. He gave me the low-cholesterol lecture, which I pretty much ignored until my follow-up physical one year later. Low and behold, my cholesterol profile worsened. Instead of starting on a medication to lower my cholesterol, I followed the Dakota Diet.

"One year later, my total cholesterol dropped from 260 to 180, my HDL [good cholesterol] went from 41 to 55 and my LDL [bad cholesterol] dropped from 148 to 110. I'd like to think that the numbers improved because I gave up french fries, but on further thought, it was based on my overall intake of food (I will not use the word *diet* here because I really did not go on a diet).

"You see, I am a big sportsman and gardener. I love to hunt and fish as well as process my catch. My freezer is full of lean meats such as buffalo, elk, and venison. My back yard garden supplied me with fresh vegetables and other ingredients for some homemade salsa and a healthy way of eating.

"So, if you have high cholesterol, try adding some venison or buffalo meat to your menu. Work in the garden, harvest your own vegetables, and go hunting! It is important for me to eat what I have hunted or harvested. I did not realize that my passion for hunting would provide me with such a healthy diet."

Homocysteine and Heart Disease

More and more, you hear of people dying of heart disease in only their third or fourth decade of life. The culprit might be high levels of an amino acid in the blood called homocysteine. Homocysteinuria occurs when your body produces abnormally high levels of homocysteine in the blood. High levels of this amino acid can actually damage the artery walls and result in cholesterol plaque formation. Just as nicotine from cigarette smoke damages the walls of arteries, high levels of homocysteine can be similarly destructive to the artery. In the body's attempt to heal itself, white blood cells (macrophages) are sent to the site of injury, carrying with them LDL cholesterol. LDLs carry most of the cholesterol to the wall of the damaged artery and are the main source of dangerous build-up and blockage in the artery. To determine if you are at risk for homocysteinuria, especially if you have a family history of heart disease, your physician will often measure your blood homocysteine level.

An easy way to prevent high levels of this amino acid is to eat foods rich in folic acid. Folic acid (or folate) is involved in a complex metabolic conversion of homocysteine to another amino acid, methionone. Other causes of elevated homocysteine include decreased absorption of folic acid by certain medications and an increased need for folic acid when taking other medications. Foods recommended on the Dakota Diet, such as legumes, green leafy vegetables, fruits, and fish, are loaded with this very important vitamin. Taking an additional vitamin B-complex, with folic acid and vitamin B_6, will also help lower your homocysteine level.

Foods Enriched with Folic Acid

Grapefruit	Asparagus	Fish	Fortified cereals
Orange juice	Broccoli	Cantaloupe	Dried beans and peas

High Blood Pressure

An estimated 50 million American adults have high blood pressure and nearly a third of those don't know they have it. Some people may experience headaches or dizziness, but for most there are no symptoms at all. High blood pressure (hypertension) can go undetected for years, damaging your tissues and vital organs. If your blood pressure is not under control, your heart may enlarge and your arteries become stiff and less elastic. Eventually, you may not be able to pump blood properly, which can lead to congestive heart failure (backup of fluid into the lungs). Damage to your arteries can trigger a heart attack, stroke, kidney disease, vision loss, and shrinkage of the brain, resulting in memory loss and dementia.

When your health-care provider measures the pressure of blood in your arteries, he or she is listening for subtle sounds generated when your heart contracts to pump blood out (your systolic pressure or the top number). Between beats, your heart fills with blood again, generating the diastolic pressure (the bottom number). A normal blood pressure is usually less than 130 (systolic) and 85 (diastolic). New blood pressure guidelines suggest that people lower this even further to around 120/80.

A high systolic pressure indicates strain on the blood vessels when the heart is attempting to pump blood into your bloodstream. If your diastolic pressure is high, it means that your blood vessels have little chance to relax between heartbeats. Having a one-time high reading does not necessarily mean you have high blood pressure, because your blood pressure varies throughout the day. In fact, it may be elevated just by the anxiety of being in the doctor's office. Your doctor will only make the diagnosis of hypertension after multiple high readings.

You may be at greater risk for high blood pressure if you have a family history of hypertension or have a pre-existing condition such as diabetes or kidney disease. Males are more prone to high blood pressure, especially African-American males. Smoking and frequent consumption of alcoholic beverages will put you at greater risk, as will obesity and living a sedentary lifestyle.

Losing as little as 10 pounds can result in a significant drop in your blood pressure. Dropping weight is by far the most effective non-drug method of lowering your blood pressure. Following the Dakota Diet can help you achieve the necessary weight loss. The Dakota Diet is also heart healthy because it is high in omega-3 fatty acids and monounsaturated fats (good fats) and contains little to none of the unhealthy fats seen in most processed foods. Several studies have shown that a diet rich in omega-3s can actually lower your blood pressure by 5 points.

A recent study found that people at risk for hypertension were able to lower their blood pressure by as much as 10–15 points by eating a diet rich in fruits, vegetables, low-fat dairy foods, and a diet low in sodium. The Dakota Diet can help you achieve this goal and also lose weight. Limiting your salt intake may be beneficial as well. Not everyone needs to restrict his or her salt, however—African Americans and women older than 65 seem to benefit the most. A reasonable limit is no more than 2,400 mg a day.

Exercise, such as 30–45 minutes of brisk walking or bike riding daily, can lower your blood pressure as well as help you burn off calories if you are trying to lose weight. Vigorous exercise for 40 minutes a day can lower your blood pressure by more than 10 points and it may keep your blood pressure down for the rest of the day. Limiting your alcohol intake may also help. Alcohol raises your blood pressure, even if you don't have hypertension; if you do have high blood pressure, it is best to avoid alcohol altogether.

If changes in eating habits and other lifestyle measures do not lower your blood pressure, then medications will be needed. Today, there are many drugs available to help lower your blood pressure and keep it under control. If your doctor prescribes high blood pressure pills, it is important that you take them every day.

There is essentially no cure for high blood pressure. However, it is both preventable and treatable. By making adjustments in your lifestyle and, if necessary, by taking medications, you can take control of your blood pressure and keep it at a safe level.

INFLAMMATORY DISEASES

A recent *Time* magazine cover story delved into the relationship between inflammation and a multitude of conditions such as cancer, Alzheimer's disease, and heart disease. Scientists have known for years how the inflammatory response to infection may lead to trauma and recent research has shown a powerful link between inflammation and a number of chronic diseases, such as arthritis, asthma, Crohn's disease, and dysmenorrhea.

To better understand how inflammation occurs when you stub your toe or get a sliver in your finger, you have to first understand the multitude of chemical reactions that occur. At the onset of injury or infection, mast cells at the site of injury immediately release the important chemical known as histamine into the area, allowing tiny blood vessels to leak, which ultimately impedes any invading bacteria. Macrophages immediately begin the counterattack by releasing cytokines into the blood, which trigger our immune system to help out. The reinforcements from our immune system help to fight off infection by destroying any bacteria at the site of injury. As a result of fighting the battle, the surrounding tissue that has been damaged by the infection or injury is destroyed as well. Eventually, the inflammatory response subsides and healing begins.

For obvious reasons, this complicated inflammatory response is a crucial first line of defense. But when this inflammatory process goes awry and does not shut down, the inflammation becomes a chronic condition affecting our health and well-being. Researchers believe that silent inflammation within the arteries of the heart causes cholesterol plaque to rupture, resulting in a heart attack. It is also believed that it is this type of inflammation that literally eats up nerve cells in the brains of Alzheimer's patients. Each one of us is getting older, and as a consequence of aging, our risk for heart disease, cancer, and Alzheimer's disease increases. What's exciting is the fact that we are now able to understand what might be taking place at the microvascular level. As research continues, newer drugs and other therapies may be developed to ward off these and other diseases common to the aging process.

Arteriosclerosis

In the 1990s, Dr. Paul Ridker, a cardiologist from Brigham Hospital, performed the initial groundbreaking research in the field of inflammation. He used a simple blood test for C-reactive protein (CRP), which is produced by the liver in response to inflammation. During active inflammation such as fighting off an infection, the CRP can be quite high. Dr. Ridker was more interested in what this protein was doing in healthy adults. To his surprise, he found that when this element was only slightly elevated, these otherwise healthy individuals were three times as likely to suffer a heart attack as those with low levels of CRP.

Physicians are only beginning to understand CRP and its part in silent inflammation. What we know of CRP is that it is an acute phase reactant, meaning that we can measure this protein through a blood sample when the body has some inflammatory activity, such as a severe infection. The level of CRP can shoot from a low of 10 mg per liter (mg/L) to 1,000 mg/L with active inflammation. Dr. Ridker and other experts determined that, in people with no outward signs of inflammation, a CRP count of greater then 3 mg/L could triple the risk of heart disease. Whereas those with a CRP count of less than 0.5 mg/L rarely suffer heart attacks.

Silent inflammation may cause plaque in the coronary artery to rupture, leading to a heart attack. As you recall, low-density lipoprotein (LDL) cholesterol is responsible for carrying cholesterol produced in the liver to the cells to be used. If you have a large number of these proteins in your body. then some of them will seep into the lining of the coronary arteries. As a result, your coronary arteries start to build up plaque within the artery, obstructing its flow. As a response to this invasion of a potentially harmful substance, your body sends macrophages (white blood cells) to the site of plaque build-up in an attempt to try to clean out the cholesterol. Cytokines (chemical messengers) are subsequently released and the inflammatory process begins. This inflammation causes the plaque to swell and rupture, resulting in clot formation and obstruction of blood flow in the artery. As a result of this blockage, your heart muscle is deprived of vital nutrients and oxygen, triggering a heart attack.

There are many risk factors that contribute to plaque rupture, including smoking, high blood pressure, and diabetes. But if there is silent inflammation going on in the body, your risk for these plaques to rupture and cause a heart attack is greater if you have high levels of CRP. This may be why many people with normal cholesterol levels end up having a heart attack. That's why the CRP test is critical for those at risk of having a stroke or heart attack.

If the LDL cholesterol level is too high in the setting of a high CRP test, then an aggressive approach to lowering cholesterol with medications, such as a statin drug, may be warranted. A statin drug can lower your LDL to less then 70 as well as lower CRP to less then 5 mg/L. Many Americans may benefit from this aggressive approach, if they can afford to pay for the prescription drugs.

The Dakota Diet can play a significant role in reducing your LDL and your risk for silent inflammation. The diet is rich in omega-3 fatty acids (found in range-fed buffalo and other foods), which balance the effects of omega-6 fatty acids. Omega-6s play a role in the production of prostaglandins responsible for inflammation in the body. In fact, a diet rich in omega-3s will act much like an aspirin does in reducing inflammation. The diet is also proven to lower your LDL levels and even raise your good (HDL) cholesterol levels. Another cause for inflammation is obesity, but the Dakota Diet is a healthy eating plan that can also help you lose any excess weight.

Rheumatoid Arthritis

Rheumatoid arthritis is an inflammatory disease afflicting over 6 million Americans. Chronic inflammation of joints and other connective tissue in the body results in the destruction of those tissues. I tell my patients that their immune system is making its own antibodies that attack the joints, causing chronic inflammation. Many patients with rheumatoid arthritis require anti-inflammatory drugs similar to aspirin to relieve their pain. Others require additional therapies that suppress the immune system from producing antibodies that destroy the joints.

Diet can play a role in squelching inflammation in the body. The Dakota Diet provides you with a balance of omega-3 to omega-6 fatty acids, so your body will produce less inflammatory acids associated with rheumatoid arthritis. Vitamin C can also play a role in preventing the development of rheumatoid arthritis. A study published in the *Annals of Rheumatic Diseases* noted that those subjects who consumed the least amounts of foods containing vitamin C were three times more likely to develop arthritis than those who consumed a diet rich in vitamin C.

Asthma

During an asthma attack, inflammatory substances known as leukotrienes are produced in the lungs. Physicians have an arsenal of medications that block the production of leukotrienes, which are eicosanoids from the omega-6 family. The omega-3 fatty acids have an opposing effect. Therefore, when eating a diet with a good ratio of omega-3 to omega-6, an asthma patient will have less of the inflammatory eicosanoids that can make asthma worse and more anti-inflammatory eicosanoids. The Dakota Diet will help you achieve this balance as you increase your consumption of food rich in omega-3s. While medications are the mainstay of asthma therapy, eating foods found in The Dakota Diet will help you achieve better asthma control.

Alzheimer's Disease

Autopsies have shown high levels of inflammatory substances known as interleukins in the brains of Alzheimer's disease sufferers. Interestingly, there are studies proving that patients with Alzheimer's disease have improved memory and mood when taking anti-inflammatory drugs. The goal in treating Alzheimer's is to reduce inflammation. This can be achieved with the right balance of omega-3 to omega-6 fatty acids. One study showed that those who ate a diet high in omega-6s had an increased incidence of dementia compared to those who consumed fish or a diet higher in omega-3s.

Chronic Obstructive Pulmonary Disease

Smoking is the leading cause of chronic obstructive pulmonary disease (COPD), in which the breathing passages and lungs are damaged by the toxins in cigarette smoke. Early signs of the disease include becoming increasingly short of breath with minimal exercise or increasing mucus production in the lungs. As the disease progresses, the ability to obtain oxygen from the air you breathe is reduced, which leads to more shortness of breath, respiratory failure, and even death.

If you smoke and are diagnosed with COPD, the obvious way to slow the progression of disease is to quit smoking. If you are exposed to secondhand smoke, you are also at risk for developing lung disease, so it is best if you can reduce your exposure. The use of steroids, either by mouth or inhaled, are a major part of the treatment of patients with COPD.

A diet with a balance of omega-3 and omega-6 fatty acids may be helpful for COPD. A large study of almost 9,000 smokers and former smokers explored the link between essential fatty acids and lung disease such as COPD. They found that those smokers who consumed a diet high in fish had a 40%–60% reduction in COPD symptoms compared to those who ate a diet with less omega-3 and more omega-6 fats. Additionally, a diet rich in vitamin A (such as the Dakota Diet) has been shown to help with lung inflammation in emphysema. Animal studies showed that rats who were vitamin A–deficient developed emphysema, but a diet rich in vitamin A helped counter this effect. Could a diet high in vitamin A explain why some smokers live into their ninth decade without significant lung disease? I am sure studies are on the way as I write.

Crohn's Disease and Ulcerative Colitis

Crohn's disease is an inflammatory condition affecting the entire gastrointestinal tract, from the mouth to the anus. The disease is manifested by abdominal pain, cramps, diarrhea, fever, and mouth ulcers, leading to weight loss and possibly even requiring surgery to remove part of the bowel that is inflamed. Crohn's disease is treated with medications that suppress the immune system, leading to a multitude of side effects. There are studies supporting a diet high in omega-3 fatty acids for keeping the disease in remission for a longer period of time.

Ulcerative colitis is another inflammatory bowel disease, which, unlike Crohn's disease, affects only the large intestine. Studies have shown that ulcerative colitis patients on medication need lower doses when they are on a diet high in omega-3 fatty acids or taking omega-3 supplements.

Lupus

Systemic lupus erythematosus (SLE) is an autoimmune disease that affects every part of the body. This disease is made worse by the typical American diet high in refined foods and omega-6 fatty acids. Studies have shown that diets rich in omega-3s helped those with SLE stay in remission for longer periods of time or use less of their medications in the treatment of the disease.

Dysmenorrhea

Dysmenorrhea is painful menstrual cramps in women. During menstruation, the body sheds the endometrial build-up in the uterus, and inflammatory prostaglandins are produced. Women who suffer from menstrual cramps typically use drugs such as ibuprofen or aspirin to block the effects of the prostaglandins. A small study of women who suffer from painful menstruation was conducted using either placebo or fish oil. Those taking fish oil (which is rich in omega-3 fatty acids) had less pain than those taking the placebo.

METABOLIC SYNDROME AND DIABETES

Has your doctor told you that you have too many fatty triglycerides in your blood and that your good cholesterol (HDL) is too low? Have you been told that the attack dogs of your arteries—the small, dense lipoproteins (very-low-density lipoproteins or VLDL)—are way too high? Then, there is the matter of your blood pressure being elevated, not to mention too much blood sugar. If you add excess abdominal fat as well as high insulin levels to the picture, then you might have a disorder called metabolic syndrome. Metabolic syndrome is actually a cluster of these risk factors, including insulin resistance, which leads to heart disease and premature death. Some researchers think metabolic syndrome may be linked to at least half of the cardiovascular disease in America today.

If your body has too much insulin (hyperinsulinemia), why is it called insulin resistance? Insulin is a hormone produced by the beta cells of the pancreas that helps maintain the proper level of glucose (sugar) in your blood. Glucose is your body's fuel—cells use it to produce energy to grow and function properly. We absorb glucose through our digestive system into the bloodstream, which then circulates the glucose to cells throughout our body. Insulin then acts like a gatekeeper, unlocking the cell to allow glucose to enter. Insulin resistance occurs when the pancreas has to secrete additional insulin in an attempt to maintain normal blood glucose. In some cases, the body cells do not respond to even high levels of insulin, keeping the gate to the cell locked, resulting in high blood glucose or type 2 diabetes. In other words, the body has more than enough insulin, but it is not producing the expected biological effect.

No one knows for sure what causes the body's cells to be resistant to its own insulin. What we do know is that insulin resistance is aggravated by obesity and physical inactivity, both of which are increasing in people of all ages in the United States. Insulin resistance seems to be the central problem of metabolic syndrome. Testing for insulin resistance is difficult and a more practical solution has yet to be developed. Until we are able to accurately test for this syndrome, researchers have determined that there are three easy measures to perform.

First, measure the fat around your middle. Some studies suggest that having a waistline over 40 inches in men and 35 inches in women may indicate the presence of metabolic syndrome. Too much abdominal visceral fat (the "beer belly") is tied to the insulin resistance syndrome. Next, obtain your total cholesterol level and divide it by your HDL (good) cholesterol level. If you are told that you have normal total cholesterol, you still may fit the metabolic syndrome profile if you have low HDL levels. A ratio greater than five points to metabolic syndrome.

The lipid profile test will also measure your LDL (bad) cholesterol level.

LDL is often within the normal range in people with metabolic syndrome. If your LDL is higher than 130, you may have heart disease unrelated to insulin resistance. Finally, determine the amount of triglycerides in your blood. Triglycerides are the small, dense lipoproteins related to what we eat or drink. The excessive calories in the foods we eat or when we drink too much alcohol turns into triglycerides. Having a large waist in combination with a low HDL level and triglycerides over 200 may indicate the presence of this deadly syndrome.

Insulin resistance is a very important risk factor for heart disease and it seems to be related to everything, including hardening of the arteries (atherosclerosis), high blood pressure, diabetes, elevated triglycerides, and clot formation. If you eat the typical American diet loaded with omega-6 fatty acids and few omega-3 fatty acids, then you are at risk for being afflicted with insulin resistance. Consuming foods high in saturated and trans-fatty acids, found in fast foods or convenience foods, puts you at additional risk for gaining weight and developing insulin resistance.

It is difficult for Americans to avoid refined carbohydrates such as candy, pastry, doughnuts, white rice, and white flour. The fast food industry has perfected the delivery of food to a busy workforce. Unfortunately, they have also fostered the perfect environment for metabolic syndrome. Refined (simple) carbohydrates such as sugar or white floor have a high glycemic index—when these refined carbohydrates are consumed, they will cause a spike in your blood sugar level. Your pancreas then has to counter the high blood glucose by secreting insulin. The cells in your body will either use the glucose as an energy source or store it in the form of fat.

Unfortunately, the cells in your body (such as muscle cells) can malfunction and not respond adequately to insulin. They essentially become resistant to normal levels of insulin, so the pancreas has to secrete more insulin to get the job done. If you continue to eat a diet with a high glycemic index, your pancreas has to pump out more and more insulin. Over time, this can burn out the pancreas. When the pancreas is no longer able to keep up with the sugars in your blood, the onset of diabetes begins and your blood glucose starts to rise.

The remedy for metabolic syndrome is simple: it is a matter of losing weight by getting regular aerobic exercise and eating right. Studies have shown that eating foods with a balance of omega-6 and omega-3 fatty acids will increase the sensitivity of your cells to insulin, thus reducing your chance of developing metabolic syndrome. Avoiding trans-fatty acids, such as margarine, will also help, because studies have shown that people who eat margarine four or more times per week were at increased risk for developing metabolic syndrome.

The Dakota Diet can help you reduce your chance of being stricken with those conditions linked to metabolic syndrome. It is a diet with a balance of omega-6 and omega-3 fatty acids. The plan also has foods with a low glycemic index that release sugar into your blood gradually, such as legumes, barley, and whole grains. I cannot stress enough the importance of maintaining an appropriate weight and being active. Many people will be able to reduce their chances of becoming insulin resistant and developing diabetes by thinking about food as a fuel for their body. Developing these long-term lifestyle changes is how to win the battle of the bulge.

Controlling Diabetes

On a daily basis, we hear of the profound effect obesity has not only on our health but on our health-care system. Despite the billions of dollars spent each year on weight loss and weight reduction products, obesity continues to be at epidemic proportions in the United States. As a result, we have over 33 million people with the type of diabetes seen in people who are overweight. Unfortunately, only about half of them know it. Type 2 diabetes is the most common form of the disease and it can develop over years, often without symptoms. It may reveal itself too late to prevent damage and many will learn they have the disease only when one of its most common complications develops—heart disease, kidney disease, or vision problems. Approximately 700,000 people are diagnosed with diabetes each year. The cost in terms of medical care, hospitalizations, time lost from work, and premature death is well over $100 billion annually.

Diabetes can lead to a group of diseases with one thing in common—a problem with insulin. The problem could be either that the body doesn't make enough (or any) insulin or that it doesn't utilize insulin properly, thus preventing the right amount of blood glucose from entering the cells. The unused glucose will build up in the blood, causing a condition known as hyperglycemia. Almost all of the symptoms of diabetes result from persistent high blood sugars. These symptoms can include frequent urination, extreme thirst, blurred vision, fatigue, unexplained weight loss, and hunger. It can also cause recurring bladder, vaginal, and skin infections, irritability, and tingling or loss of feeling in the hands or feet. Diseases associated with diabetes can affect almost every major part of the body. Diabetes can result in blindness, heart disease, strokes, kidney failure, amputations, nerve damage, and birth defects in babies born to women with diabetes.

Type 2 diabetes usually develops after the age of 40 and is more common among American Indians, Hispanics, and African Americans. If you have a family history of diabetes, your risk is increased. Unfortunately, being overweight at any age will put you at risk for developing diabetes. In fact, doctors once classified diabetes as "adult onset" or "juvenile onset" diabetes, but now adult-onset diabetes is commonly seen as a result of over-eating and inactivity in children.

Obesity is by far the greatest risk factor—80% to 90% of type 2 diabetics are overweight, which increases insulin resistance. The pancreas is essentially called upon to produce more insulin, and if it cannot keep up, blood sugar begins to rise. Losing weight will allow you to achieve normal blood sugar levels without the use of expensive medications, which may have undesirable side effects. Achieving and maintaining a healthy weight is extremely beneficial, especially when combined with exercise. Exercise not only reduces insulin resistance, it also improves your body's ability to tolerate elevated blood sugars. If you are prone to diabetes, you can cut your risk in half with regular exercise as well as losing and maintaining your weight.

How much you eat is as important as what you eat in reducing the risk for diabetes. The amount of food you consume will ultimately determine your weight, and being overweight significantly increases your risk. If you are a diabetic, eating large amounts of high-glycemic foods or simple carbohydrates will push your blood sugar higher, and skipping meals may cause it to fall too low (hypoglycemia). To prevent these glucose swings, eat smaller servings at regular intervals. Foods of the Dakota Diet, such as whole grains, legumes, fruits, and vegetables, are high in fiber and have a low glycemic index. You can control these blood sugar swings by eating these types of foods.

Diabetics are at a higher risk for heart disease; so they should keep their dietary fat consumption at around 35% of their total daily calories. The foods you eat should be low in saturated fat, trans-fatty acids, and omega-6 fatty acids but relatively high in omega-3s and unsaturated oils. Recent studies support a diet favoring omega-3s and unsaturated fats (as seen in the Dakota Diet)—diabetics on this type of diet have better sensitivity to insulin, an improved cholesterol profile, lower triglycerides, and lower blood pressure.

If you have diabetes, controlling your blood sugar is the single most important thing you can do to prevent disease. I cannot stress enough the importance of a healthy diet along with weight loss and exercise as key elements in the treatment and control of type 2 diabetes. If that approach alone isn't successful, your doctor may prescribe medications in addition to diet and exercise to maintain a normal blood sugar level. Today, living with diabetes does not necessarily mean a drastic change in your lifestyle. By following a few healthy guidelines—eating the right foods, watching your weight, not smoking, and getting regular exercise—most diabetics can enjoy an active lifestyle and live a normal life span.

CANCER

Prostate Cancer

A diet low in saturated fat and rich in omega-3 fatty acids has been shown to reduce serum testosterone levels in men with prostate cancer. A study published in *Lancet* suggested that consuming foods rich in omega-3s, such as fatty fish (trout and salmon), will not only help reduce or prevent heart disease, it may even prevent cancer in men. Men who ate no fish were two to three times more likely to develop prostate cancer than those who ate a moderate amount of fish. Another study published in *Urology* showed a slower growth rate of cancer cells as well as an increase in prostate cancer cell death when men consumed ground flaxseed, which is high in omega-3s and lignan, a phytoestrogen that inhibits prostate cancer formation and growth. These plant-derived estrogens may actually interfere with the conversion of testosterone to the more potent hormone known as dihydrotestosterone (DHT). The Dakota Diet is a great way to take advantage of these findings.

Colon Cancer

Colon cancer strikes nearly 135,000 Americans per year and is the nation's second-highest cause of cancer deaths, killing over 55,000 people a year. Tragically for many patients, a delay in diagnosis is the primary reason for the advanced stage of the disease at presentation and is associated with a poor outcome. Regular screening can detect many of these cancers at an earlier stage that is more favorable for treatment. A fair amount of colon cancer cases occur in families—if a first-degree relative (parent, sibling, or child) has either a colon polyp or cancer, you may be genetically predisposed to cancer of the colon.

You can lower your risk for developing colon cancer by eating plenty of raw fruits and vegetables and by limiting your intake of highly saturated fats. Consuming foods rich in omega-3s, vitamin D, and calcium (such as are found in the Dakota Diet) may also lower your colon cancer risk. Studies of Eskimos whose diet consists mainly of fish rich in omega-3 fatty acids, show a lower rate of colon cancer.

Breast Cancer

Breast cancer is the most common cancer in women, with more than 210,000 new cases diagnosed in the United States each year. One in seven American women (13%) will develop breast cancer in her lifetime. Studies have shown that obesity, especially in menopausal women, and a diet high in saturated fat may have an impact on the development of breast cancer. Breast cancer is less common in countries where the typical diet is low in total fat. Researchers believe that a diet rich in omega-3 fatty acids along with important antioxidants such as vitamin C and E, beta-carotene, and selenium (all found in the Dakota Diet) may help prevent breast cancer. More research is needed to gain a better understanding of the health impact of dietary fats and body weight on the risk for developing breast cancer.

EYE DISEASES

Macular Degeneration

The most common cause of vision loss in the elderly is an age-related disease known as macular degeneration. It occurs when part of the retina (the layer of tissue on the inside back wall of the eyeball) known as the macula starts to deteriorate, resulting in blurred vision or a blind spot in the center of the visual field. A 2004 study published in the *Archives of Ophthalmology* showed that eating three or more servings of fruit per day will lower the risk of developing macular degeneration. Consuming fruits rich in vitamins A, C, and E, and the carotenoid lutein provided protection from macular degeneration. Studies have shown that people who had a healthy dietary balance of omega-3 and omega-6 fatty acids are less likely to develop this illness. You can get these benefits from following the Dakota Diet.

Cataracts

A cataract is a collection of dead cells that accumulate in the lens of the eye. The lens is responsible for focusing light and producing clear, sharp images. Over time, the cataract causes the lens to cloud, making images look blurred or fuzzy. Cataracts can be a part of the natural aging process; however, the damaging ultraviolet rays from the sun will accelerate the process. Fruits and vegetables containing carotenoids help protect the eyes from the damaging effects of ultraviolet light from the sun. Lutein is an important carotenoid that is abundant in foods such as kale and spinach. One study noted that people who eat foods rich in lutein had a 50% reduced risk for developing cataracts. Because lutein is fat-soluble, fat is needed in the diet in order to absorb lutein from the diet. I would recommend using a little olive oil on your kale or spinach in order to maximize lutein absorption.

OSTEOPOROSIS

Of the estimated 50 million people over the age of 50, half are afflicted by osteoporosis. The difference between bone loss attributed to the natural aging process and bone loss due to osteoporosis is significant. In post-menopausal osteoporosis, the rate of bone loss exceeds the rate of bone formation. When bone formation cannot catch up to bone loss, osteoporosis sets in. The primary cause for osteoporosis is advancing age, which is spurred by a decline in the hormone estrogen.

Preventing bone loss is more practical then treating bone loss. To reduce bone loss and increase bone mass, a woman needs to consume approximately 1,000–1,500 mg of calcium a day. Eight ounces of skim milk contains

300 mg of calcium as does 8 ounces of calcium-fortified orange juice, 1-$\frac{1}{2}$ cups of steamed broccoli, or about 6 ounces of salmon. Supplements are useful for those who can't increase their calcium intake through diet. Vitamin D (400 IU) as well as adequate amounts of vitamin C and protein are important to prevent further bone loss. Deficiencies in these nutrients can affect the bone mass. A diet rich in omega-3 fatty acids with less omega-6 fatty acids has been shown to prevent osteoporosis in both men and women. Weight-bearing exercise, in the form of walking, aids in conserving bone density and helps to maintain flexibility and muscle strength.

IRRITABLE BOWEL SYNDROME

If you have ever had problems with abdominal pain and abnormal bowel movements, you may be suffering symptoms of irritable bowel syndrome (IBS). As many as 20% to 40% of the American population experiences symptoms similar to yours. IBS is due to an abnormality in the function of the intestines, without structural damage or disease. The colon (large bowel) seems to be the major part of the intestine that is affected. Its normal function is to absorb water and minerals from the bowel contents as it propels them along. In IBS, the movements of the colon are abnormal, leading to diarrhea, constipation, and abdominal pain related to spasm of the colon or due to distention from trapped gas. This does not mean that the colon is damaged or diseased, which is why x-rays and other tests are typically normal in patients with irritable bowel.

Unfortunately, research in this area has been limited. For years, IBS was thought to be a psychosomatic illness, with all the symptoms being related to stress. What we do know about irritable bowel is that there are a number of factors (including stress) that aggravate the colon, including sensitivity to certain foods such as fatty or greasy foods, coffee, and alcohol. IBS is very much like migraine headaches—a true medical illness that is not purely psychosomatic or stress related, but one which may be triggered by stress. Some patients have their worst symptoms when they are doing their best in terms of dealing with the stresses in their lives. Others find that the symptoms are worse either during severe stress or immediately following an episode of stress.

When irritable bowel symptoms are infrequent, no treatment is necessary other than reassurance. In some cases, symptoms of diarrhea or pain are normal responses to stress and will therefore be resolved when the stress is gone. Many patients with IBS are found to be lactose intolerant and should avoid milk and other dairy products. A high-fiber diet, as seen in the Dakota Diet, will often control symptoms in as many as two-thirds of those with irritable bowel.

MOOD DISORDERS

The brain is a fatty organ, with up to 60% of the mass of the brain composed of fat. Research is now showing a link between mood disorders, such as depression, bipolar disorder, dementia, and even schizophrenia, and a lack of omega-3 fatty acids. Clinical trials using omega-3s are under way to look at their usefulness in helping to regulate mental disorders. In the meantime, increasing omega-3 levels in the diet might be helpful.

Studies suggest that those who have a diet high in omega-3 fatty acids are less likely to experience feelings of depression or hostility. Researchers believe that those people who do not get enough omega-3 fatty acids in their diet are at risk for depression. Omega-3s are essential for maintaining mental health because they may help keep patterns of thought and mental reactions running smoothly and efficiently in the brain. Those with bipolar disorder (also known as manic-depressive disorder) may benefit from a diet higher in omega-3 fats as well. One study showed that those who were treated with omega-3 supplements, in addition to their medications, experienced fewer mood swings than those who received nothing at all.

Attention Deficit Disorder (ADD)

An estimated 3% to 5% of school-age children (3.5 million) have attention deficit disorder (ADD). Purdue University conducted a study of boys with low levels of omega-3 fatty acids. They had a greater tendency of problems with learning and behavior consistent with ADD. Animal studies have also shown that low levels of omega-3 fatty acids were correlated to a lower concentration of other substances in the brain such as dopamine and serotonin, which are important neurochemicals related to attention and motivation. At the present time, there are no studies to support the use of omega-3 supplements to improve symptoms of ADD. However, I would suggest that a diet high in omega-3s is a healthier diet for anyone, including children with a diagnosis of ADD.

FIBROMYALGIA

You wake up in the morning and hurt all over. Your muscles are stiff and you find it difficult to get out of bed. You are constantly fatigued and have difficulty sleeping. You seek medical advice from all types of health-care providers, yet no one can give you a definitive diagnosis for what ails you. If you are experiencing these symptoms, you might be suffering from a condition called fibromyalgia.

Approximately 7–10 million Americans suffer from this disorder, which is characterized by chronic pain in the muscles, ligaments, and tendons. It is often called fibromyalgia syndrome, meaning that it is not a specific illness but a condition that involves several symptoms that occur together. Fibromyalgia is often associated with difficulty sleeping, stress, anxiety, depression, headaches, tingling in your hands and feet, and digestive problems. The symptoms may come and go but they never completely disappear. Although it tends to be a chronic condition, fibromyalgia syndrome isn't progressive, crippling, or life-threatening.

Medical science has yet to find a cause or cure for fibromyalgia. There are many theories, but none has been proven. One theory is that certain factors such as stress, poor sleep, physical or emotional trauma, or being out of shape may trigger the condition in people who are more sensitive to pain.

Diagnosing fibromyalgia can be challenging, because there isn't a single test that can confirm or rule out the condition. People with fibromyalgia often go through several medical tests only to have the results turn up normal—yet their pain is real. When a physician has ruled out other conditions that may mimic fibromyalgia, such as a thyroid disorder or rheumatoid arthritis, a diagnosis of fibromyalgia is made. The American College of Rheumatology has established some general guidelines for diagnosing fibromyalgia, including whole-body aching for at least three months and a minimum of 11 body locations (called trigger points) that are painfully tender under mild pressure.

Fibromyalgia syndrome patients should maintain a healthy diet, as seen in the Dakota Diet, and eliminate inflammatory foods such as refined foods, sugars, and saturated fat. Consuming foods rich in omega-3 fatty acids may aid in the reduction of symptoms. There's no known cure for fibromyalgia, but a comprehensive approach may be helpful.

Developing a plan to avoid or limit the stress in your life is essential. Allow yourself some time each day to relax, but don't change your routine totally. People who quit work or drop all activity tend to do worse than those who remain active. Try to exercise at least 20 to 30 minutes a day, three times a week. At first, exercise may increase your pain, but doing it regularly often improves symptoms. Keep your activity on an even level. If you do too much on your good days, you may have more bad days. If you are deconditioned, you should start out with just 3–5 minutes of exercise every day and increase as tolerated. Avoid exercising the most painful muscles.

Getting adequate sleep is essential, because fibromyalgia symptoms often appear during times of sleep disruption. Working night shifts or having to get up to attend to your children will fragment your sleep and make your symptoms worse. Re-establishing a regular sleep schedule may be enough to relieve your symptoms. Your physician may also prescribe medications to help improve your sleep: they should be started at the lowest possible dose and increased slowly so that you get maximum relief of daytime symptoms without unacceptable side effects.

Some people get relief from massages, hot baths, and relaxation techniques. Other complementary therapies include myofascial release therapy, water therapy, light aerobics, acupressure, aromatherapy, biofeedback, breathing techniques, and many more. Most patients can be helped with a combination of medications, exercise, and maintaining a regular sleep schedule. Making these lifestyle changes can relieve fibromyalgia symptoms or even make them disappear.

Conclusion

In America, the word *diet* or *dieting* can evoke a number of bad feelings. Many of us have tried a diet, yet failed to lose the necessary weight or gained back what we lost and possibly more. Most of the popular diets are nearly impossible to follow, let alone maintain for any length of time. On the other hand, when we use the word *diet* in the phrase "healthy diet," we tend to believe that the foods involved are inaccessible or undesirable.

Not so with the Dakota Diet. This book was written for the sole purpose of providing the reader with information on how nutrition can affect one's health and even prevent disease. I like to consider the Dakota Diet as a healthy lifestyle rather than just a diet. The foods discussed in this book can be grown in any garden or come from animals found ranging free on grasslands throughout the country. The nutrients in these foods and animals of the Dakotas are healthier.

The health implications of being obese are stark and clear. If you are overweight, you are at risk for just about every disease I describe in this book. Having an understanding of what can happen to the body as a result of these diseases will empower you to take action for your own health.

Whether you hunt, garden, shop the farmers markets, or buy organics, the food you eat can make a difference in your health. Start now by eating the right foods, eating less of them, and continuing to burn more calories. Start now for a healthier you!

The Dakota Diet

APPENDIX A

Chefs of the Dakotas and Their Recipes

After spending our third and fourth years of medical school in the Black Hills of South Dakota, my wife and I not only fell in love with each other but also with the land and its hardworking people. You have to love where you live, and the Black Hills have given us the opportunity to explore the Wild West, as well as enjoy some of the finest foods, right here in our back yard.

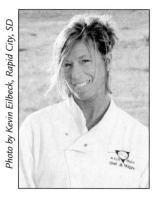

Photo by Kevin Eilbeck, Rapid City, SD

Jill Maguire

Wild Idea Buffalo Company
P.O. Box 1209
Rapid City, SD 57709-1209
Web site: www.wildideabuffalo.com

We're fortunate to have met chef Jill Maguire, who has had several restaurants in the area, including Sweet Grass Buffalo Grill, located near the historic town of Deadwood, South Dakota. She currently owns and operates Wild Idea Buffalo Company and has become a culinary expert with bison meat. "The food industry is constantly changing and although the finished product is the ultimate goal, it's the quality and consistency of the original product that determines your success," says Jill. "Wild Idea Buffalo meat will certainly add to the success of your meal, not just in taste, but also in the health benefits it offers, no matter what the trend." She is currently working on a cookbook and has included several of her buffalo recipes for the Dakota Diet.

Grilled Bison Steak

Bison steaks
Garlic salt
Pepper
Cooking oil
Lemon pepper

Rub your favorite 6-ounce cut of bison steak with a combination of a little garlic salt, pepper, cooking oil, and lemon pepper. Grill steaks for the following times, depending on thickness. Precise cooking time is important in order to avoid overcooking. Times reflect total cooking time (both sides).

- 1-inch thick steak: rare, 6–8 minutes; medium, 8–10 minutes.

- $1\frac{1}{2}$-inch thick steak: rare, 8–10 minutes; medium, 10–12 minutes.

- 2-inch thick steak: rare: 10–12 minutes; medium, 14–18 minutes.

Rib eyes, T-bones, and New York strips are the best for grilling or barbecuing. I find that steaks taste best when grilled rare to medium rare (still pink in the center). The lesser quality steaks are not recommended for grilling unless they have been marinated.

Buffalo Osso Bucco

YIELD: 4 servings

4 buffalo shanks
4 tbsp olive oil
$\frac{1}{4}$ cup flour
1 tsp salt and pepper
1 onion, sliced
1 tbsp garlic
Sprigs fresh thyme
1 bottle white wine
Zest of lemon
$\frac{1}{2}$ cup parsley

Season shanks with salt and pepper. Dredge shanks in a mixture of flour, salt, and pepper. Brown the floured shanks in olive oil in a deep skillet on medium-high heat. Add onions, thyme, and garlic after you have turned the shanks. De glaze pan with wine and bring to boil (see next recipe for De Glaze). Reduce heat to simmer and continue to slow cook for 2 hours. Remove the shanks from the pan and reduce the juices. Add lemon zest and parsley. Pour sauce over shanks and serve.

Buffalo Roast with Au Jus

YIELD: 4 to 6 servings

3-pound buffalo sirloin tip or top round roast

$\frac{1}{2}$ onion or $\frac{1}{2}$ celery stalk

Olive oil

Salt & pepper

Herb Paste:

1 tsp each thyme, sage, salt, pepper

1 tbsp garlic, chopped

1 tbsp olive oil

1 tbsp balsamic vinegar

De glaze sauce:

$\frac{1}{3}$ cup red wine

$\frac{1}{8}$ cup Madeira wine

$\frac{3}{4}$ cup beef stock

Preheat oven to 475°F. Place seasoned roast in a roasting pan on a bed of onions or celery. Sear in a hot oven for 10 minutes. Reduce the temperature to 350°F. Add $\frac{1}{2}$ cup of water to bottom of the pan and brush the roast with herb paste. Continue this process every 10 minutes until internal temperature reaches 130°F (about 30 to 40 minutes).

Remove roast and vegetables from pan. Place roasting pan on stove top on medium-high burner. De glaze. Scrape bottom of pan and reduce to half. Slice roast and serve with Au jus.

Buffalo Burgers

YIELD: 6 patties

2 pounds ground buffalo

2 tbsp olive oil

$\frac{1}{2}$ tsp mustard

1 tsp ketchup

1 tsp thyme

1 tsp Worcestershire sauce

2 tsp salt & pepper

Mix all ingredients but buffalo into a paste. Pour on the buffalo and mix thoroughly with hands. Make into six patties. Return to the refrigerator to allow the burgers to firm up. Then, spray outside with olive oil and season with garlic pepper. Grill for 3 to 4 minutes on each side for medium rare. Finish with a sprinkle of high-quality salt before serving.

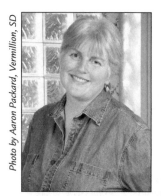

Photo by Aaron Packard, Vermillion, SD

Virginia Koster

Emma's Kitchen

13 West Main Street

Vermillion, SD 57069

Phone: 605-624-9337

Chef Virginia Koster (known as "The Prairie Gourmet" to those who have listened to South Dakota public broadcasting) shows us her ability to prepare lamb as well as other Midwest cuisines. She perfected her skills working with author and chef Nancy Verde Barr as well as with chef Bruce Tillinghast, of Providence, Rhode Island. She believes that home cooks should "relax and enjoy the time in the kitchen and that recipes should be treated as guides rather than gospel, to be generous with flavors, inquisitive and experimental, and to serve everything with a dash of love."

Barley Salad with Shallot Vinaigrette

YIELD: 6 servings

1 cup pearled barley

$\frac{1}{2}$ cup dried currants

$\frac{1}{2}$ cup sliced red onion

2 cups cooked soybeans (frozen sweet soybeans)

1 red bell pepper, finely chopped

2 stalks celery, thinly sliced on diagonal

$\frac{1}{2}$ cup parsley, chopped

Vinaigrette:

2 shallots, peeled and minced

$\frac{1}{2}$ cup white wine vinegar

1 tbsp sugar

$\frac{1}{4}$ cup canola oil

1–2 tsp Kosher salt, to taste

1 tsp freshly ground black pepper

Rinse barley and put in a saucepan, cover with 4 cups of boiling water, and let sit for 1 hour. Place saucepan on heat and cook barley, stirring occasionally, for about 15–20 minutes, until soft but still chewy. Drain in a colander and rinse briefly with cold water.

In a large mixing bowl, add the currants, onion, soybeans, pepper, celery, and parsley. In a small bowl or measuring cup, mix all the vinaigrette ingredients and whisk to combine. Add the dressing to the bowl of vegetables and toss. Then, add the barley and toss all ingredients until mixed well. Taste and adjust seasonings—you may need more salt and pepper. Serve as a side dish or main lunch course on a bed of greens.

Curried Red Lentil Soup

YIELD: **6 servings**

3 tbsp canola oil

4 garlic cloves, minced

Fresh ginger root (2-inch piece, peeled, and minced or grated)

1 cup onions, finely chopped

1 cup carrots, finely chopped

1 cup celery, finely chopped

1 red bell pepper, finely chopped

1 tbsp curry powder

1 tsp ground coriander

1 tsp cumin seeds, crushed or ground

$\frac{1}{2}$ tsp cinnamon

Salt and freshly ground black pepper

For extra heat, add $\frac{1}{2}$ tsp (or more) crushed red pepper flakes

6 cups water or vegetable broth

1 cup red lentils, washed and sorted

Zest and juice of 1 lime

1 handful fresh cilantro, chopped

Garnish: additional chopped fresh cilantro
and non- or low-fat plain yogurt

In a 4–6 quart stockpot with a heavy bottom, cook garlic, ginger, and onions in the canola oil over medium heat, stirring frequently, until the onions are soft and translucent. Season with a little salt while stirring. Do not brown (turn heat lower if necessary). Because of the small amount of oil, you may need to add a dash of water now and then to keep the vegetables from sticking.

Add the chopped carrots and celery and stir for 1–2 minutes longer. Add chopped red pepper, and stir briefly. Then, add the spices to the pot and stir to combine with the vegetables. Continue to cook over low-medium heat, stirring frequently for about 2 more minutes. Add 6 cups of water or vegetable broth and red lentils to the pot. Stir and raise the heat to high and bring the mixture to a boil. Reduce heat to simmer and cook the soup until the lentils are tender, about 20 minutes. When the lentils are soft and breaking apart and the soup has thickened, it is ready.

Add the zest and juice of 1 lime and a handful of chopped fresh cilantro to the pot, stir and adjust seasonings. You may wish to add a little salt and freshly ground black pepper, to taste, at this time. Ladle into individual bowls and garnish with a dollop of yogurt and additional chopped fresh cilantro.

Heart Soup

YIELD: *2 servings*

¼ cup extra-virgin olive oil

1 small onion, peeled and chopped

2 cloves garlic, peeled and sliced thin

½ tsp crushed red pepper flakes

1 tbsp fresh rosemary leaves

2 cups chicken or vegetable broth

1 15-oz can chickpeas, drained

1–2 tbsp fresh lemon juice

1 large roasted red pepper, peeled

1 tbsp fresh lemon juice

½ clove garlic, pressed

Salt and freshly ground black pepper to taste

Garnishes: *extra-virgin olive oil and fresh parsley*

In a 1–2 quart saucepan with a heavy bottom, heat olive oil and add onion and garlic. Stir over medium heat until onions are soft and translucent. Add salt, pepper, red pepper flakes, and rosemary and stir to incorporate. Add broth, drained chickpeas, and lemon juice and bring to a boil. Reduce heat and simmer for about 10 minutes. Puree the chickpea soup in a blender or food processor.

While the soup is simmering, put the pepper, lemon juice, pressed garlic, and salt and pepper in a blender or small food processor. Process until it becomes a thick, smooth, bright red mixture.

To serve, ladle the chickpea soup into two shallow soup bowls. Using a spoon, gently lay two scoops of the pepper mixture in the center of the bowl to make a heart shape. Garnish soup with a "squiggle" of extra-virgin olive oil and a few parsley leaves.

Romantic Dinner for Two with Lamb Chops

4 small lamb chops
(about 1 ½ inches thick)

2 garlic cloves, minced

1 tbsp chopped fresh rosemary

Lemon-Mustard Dressing/Marinade
(recipe follows)

2 fresh beets, peeled, washed, and shredded
(using a sharp grater or food processor)

¼ cup chopped, fresh herbs
(parsley, scallions, cilantro, etc.)

Baby greens

Mashed potatoes

Kosher salt and freshly ground black pepper

Rub garlic and rosemary onto both sides of each lamb chop. Place chops on a plate and pour about 2 tbsp of Lemon-Mustard Dressing/Marinade over the chops to coat evenly. Let stand for about 30 minutes.

Mix several tablespoons of Lemon-Mustard Dressing/Marinade with shredded beets and herbs and set aside.

Meanwhile, heat a heavy frying pan (cast iron, if possible) over high heat. The pan should be lightly coated with olive oil. When the pan is very hot, shake any loose dressing off the lamb chops and place them in the pan. Fry the chops for 2–3 minutes per side for rare to medium-rare, or to taste.

Prepare two dinner plates with a mound of baby greens; arrange shredded beet salad on greens next to a mound of mashed potatoes. (Use a heart-shaped cookie cutter to shape the beets and potatoes on the greens.) Remove chops from the heat, and arrange two lamb chops over beets and potatoes on each dinner plate. Sprinkle each entrée with Lemon-Mustard Dressing/Marinade and garnish with fresh herbs.

(For heart-healthy mashed potatoes, instead of using butter and cream, mash potatoes with low-fat milk, extra-virgin olive oil, and a bit of prepared horseradish and pressed garlic, salt, and pepper. Chopped fresh chives and/or parsley will add extra flavor.)

Lemon-Mustard Dressing/Marinade (2 servings):

Zest of 1 lemon

¼ cup fresh lemon juice

2 garlic cloves, pressed

1 tbsp coarse Dijon mustard

1 tsp Kosher salt

Freshly ground black pepper

½ tsp sugar

¼ cup extra-virgin olive oil

¼ cup canola oil

In a bowl, combine all ingredients except oils with a whisk. Then, add the oils in a slow stream while whisking. Use this dressing for greens, beet salad, and as a marinade for lamb or beef. The dressing will keep for several days in the refrigerator.

Mediterranean Lamb Stew

Yield: 4 to 6 servings

¼ cup extra-virgin olive oil

1½ to 2 pounds boneless leg of lamb (in 1-inch cubes)

4 cloves garlic, minced

2 medium yellow onions, chopped

Salt and freshly ground black pepper to taste

2–3 cups fresh Italian parsley, chopped

Juice of 2 large fresh lemons, divided

1 small can of tomato paste

1 cup chicken or beef stock

2–3 cups cooked chickpeas

Garnish: *fresh parsley and extra-virgin olive oil*

In a heavy, ovenproof pot, heat olive oil over high heat, then add lamb cubes and brown. Add garlic, onion, salt, and pepper. Stir and cook over medium heat until onions begin to soften. Add parsley, juice of 1 lemon, tomato paste, and stock and mix together. Cover pot with cooking parchment and a lid, or some foil over the top. Place in 350°F oven and bake for 1 ½ to 2 hours, or until lamb is very tender.

If the stew becomes dry during cooking, add more water, lemon juice, or stock to the pan. When the lamb is cooked tender, add the chickpeas, stir, and bake another few minutes until heated through. Taste and adjust seasonings; add more lemon juice to taste. The stew should be tart. Garnish with fresh parsley and a sprinkle of extra-virgin olive oil and freshly ground black pepper. Serve with orzo noodles, rice, or pita bread.

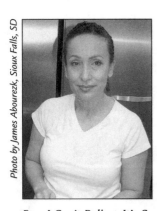

Photo by James Abourezk, Sioux Falls, SD

Sanaa Abourezk

Sanaa's Gourmet Mediterranean
401 E. 8th Street, #100
Sioux Falls, SD 57103
Web site: www.sanaasgourmet.com

Author, nutritionist, and chef Sanaa Abourezk knows the right blend of herbs and spices, bringing the art of cooking soy to another level in her book *Oh Boy, I Can't Believe It's Soy.* Sanaa believes that soy should not only taste good, it should also "provide nourishment and enrich the body." Having a degree in agricultural engineering as well as a Master's degree in nutrition gives her book on cooking soy a lot of credibility. Additionally, her skills as a chef were honed at the Masha Innocenti Cooking School, in Florence, Italy, as well as the Cordon Bleu, in Paris, France. Many of her healthy cuisines can be enjoyed at Sanaa's Gourmet Mediterranean Restaurant in Sioux Falls, South Dakota.

Acorn Squash Soup

YIELD: 4 servings

1 tbsp olive oil

3 oz leek, chopped

6 oz acorn squash, peeled and cut into 1-inch cubes

1 small yam, peeled and cut into 1-inch cubes

4 cups water, divided

6 oz lite tofu, drained

$\frac{1}{8}$ tsp nutmeg

2 cloves

$\frac{1}{8}$ tsp curry powder

1 cube vegetable bouillon

Salt to taste

Sauté the leeks in olive oil over low heat for a couple of minutes Add the rest of vegetables plus $\frac{1}{4}$ cup of water and continue to cook for 5 minutes, stirring occasionally. Add the tofu, seasonings, vegetable bouillion cube, and the rest of the water and cook over low to medium heat until the vegetables are soft. Remove the cloves, then puree the soup in a food processor or blender until smooth. Return to the pot. Add water if the soup is too thick. Adjust the seasonings and cook over low heat for 5 minutes, then serve.

Bean Curry

YIELD: 4 servings

8 oz lite tofu, drained

1 medium onion, julienned

1 tbsp olive oil

2 cloves garlic, mashed

$\frac{1}{2}$ tbsp curry powder

2 cups water

2 cups boiled soybeans

Salt to taste

Cut tofu into 1-inch cubes. Sauté onions in oil for a couple of minutes. Add the garlic and curry, stir, and cook over low heat for 1 minute. Add water and bring to a boil. Then, add beans and seasoning. Boil over medium heat for 5 minutes. Adjust seasonings, and add tofu cubes. Stir carefully and simmer over low heat for 10 minutes. Serve with steamed rice or your choice of pasta.

Tofu Lasagna

YIELD: *8 servings*

12 oz lite tofu

$\frac{1}{4}$ cup soy milk

$\frac{1}{2}$ cup Parmesan cheese, divided

6 cloves garlic

10 fresh basil leaves, chopped

2 tbsp olive oil

salt

15 lasagna noodles

4 cups tomato sauce

In a food processor, puree the tofu, soy milk, cheese, garlic, basil, oil, and salt to a smooth paste (pesto sauce).

In a large pan, bring salted water to a boil. Add the lasagna noodles and cook until al dente. Remove and place on a dish towel to cool. Grease a 13" x 9" baking dish. Pour a thin layer of tomato sauce on the bottom of dish and cover with three noodles. Spread a generous amount of tomato sauce over first layers of noodles. Cover tomato sauce with another three noodles. Cover second layer of noodles with a generous amount of pesto sauce. Repeat, in order, until you have five layers with tomato sauce over the last layer.

Cover with foil and bake at 400°F for 25 minutes. Remove foil and continue to bake for another 10 minutes, then serve.

Angel Hair Pasta Mold

YIELD: *6 servings*

12 oz lite tofu, drained and pureed

4 cloves garlic

1 cup Parmesan cheese, divided

$\frac{1}{4}$ cup chopped fresh basil leaves

2 tbsp olive oil

salt to taste

1 pound angel hair pasta

$\frac{1}{4}$ cup bread crumbs

In a food processor, puree tofu, garlic, $\frac{1}{2}$ cup of cheese, basil, olive oil, and salt to a smooth paste. In a large pot, bring salted water to boil. Add the pasta and cook until al dente; drain. Add the pasta while it is hot to the tofu paste and mix well until all pasta is coated with the tofu paste. Mix the rest of the cheese with the bread crumbs. Spray a cake pan with olive oil spray, then coat the pan with half of the cheese and bread crumbs mixture. Stuff the cake pan with the pasta, pressing it very firmly into the cake pan. Sprinkle the top with the rest of the cheese and crumb mixture. Bake in a 375°F oven for 35 minutes. Serve with mixed salad.

ADDITIONAL RECIPES

Blueberry Flax Pancakes

YIELD: *12 pancakes (4 servings)*

2 cups of all-purpose baking mix

$1\frac{1}{2}$ cups skim milk

1 free-range or cage-free egg

$\frac{3}{4}$ tsp ground cinnamon

1 cup ground flaxseed

1 cup blueberries

Mix all ingredients except blueberries until blended, then fold in the blueberries. On a hot griddle coated with non-stick spray, pour $\frac{1}{3}$ cup of batter for each pancake. Flip when the pancake bubbles through and becomes dry around the edges. If the batter is too thick, add some extra milk.

Bison Kebobs

YIELD: 4 servings

1 pound sirloin

2 medium zucchini or yellow squash

1 large red bell pepper

1 large onion, quartered

8 mushrooms

8 cherry tomatoes

Marinade:

$\frac{1}{2}$ cup low-sodium soy sauce

$\frac{1}{2}$ cup canola oil

1 cup dry white wine

2 cloves garlic, minced

The sirloin should be cut into $1\frac{1}{2}$-inch cubes and marinated in the refrigerator for 12–24 hours. The squash and bell pepper should be cut into $\frac{1}{2}$-inch pieces. Skewer the meat and vegetables as desired and grill over medium-hot coals for 8–10 minutes, brushing with marinade occasionally.

Grilled Buffalo Ribs

YIELD: 2 to 3 servings

3 pounds buffalo (or beef) ribs

3 tbsp garlic, pureed

2 tbsp fresh rosemary, chopped ($\frac{3}{4}$ tablespoon dried)

2 tbsp fresh thyme, chopped ($\frac{3}{4}$ tablespoon dried)

$1\frac{1}{2}$ tsp coarse salt

1 tbsp cracked black pepper

Pat dry the ribs with paper towels. Mix garlic, rosemary, thyme, and salt and coat ribs. Sprinkle with pepper, then refrigerate for 1 hour. Adjust grill to 6 inches above coals or grill over medium-low heat for 45 minutes, turning frequently.

Deer/Venison Chili

YIELD: 6 to 8 servings

1 1/2 pounds dry red beans

1 1/2 gallons hot water

7 cloves garlic, peeled and diced to a pulp

1/2 large onion, diced

1/3 cup of olive oil or canola oil

2 pounds coarse ground venison

1/2 cup chili powder

1/3 cup salt (if you have a history of high blood pressure,
add salt to taste or salt substitute)

3 tbsp black pepper

1/2 tsp cayenne pepper (optional)

Add the red beans to the hot water; bring to boil and cook until tender (approximately 40 minutes). Add garlic, onion, and olive or canola oil to the ground meat. Brown mixture until completely cooked (approximately 20 minutes). Add the remaining spices and seasonings to the cooked meat. When beans are tender, add meat and stir thoroughly.

Deer/Venison Roast

YIELD: 4 to 6 servings

1 clove garlic, diced to a pulp

1/2 tsp marjoram

1 tsp salt

1/2 tsp black pepper

1/2 cup of canola oil

1 (3-pound) roast of venison

Add garlic and other seasonings to the oil and let stand for 30 minutes. Preheat oven to 350°F. With a pastry brush, coat the roast on all sides with the oil and seasonings. Bake for 25–30 minutes per pound. Baste often.

Glazed Deer/Venison Meatloaf

YIELD: 6 to 8 servings

Red Currant Glaze:

$\frac{1}{2}$ large onion, diced.

2 ribs celery, diced

1 tsp salt (optional or to taste)

$\frac{1}{2}$ tsp pepper

2 pounds ground venison

2 beef bouillon cubes

$\frac{1}{2}$ cup hot water

3 omega-3-enriched eggs

$\frac{3}{4}$ cup whole-wheat cracker meal

Olive or Canola oil

Red Currant Glaze:

$\frac{1}{4}$ cup red currant jelly

1 tbsp Crème de Cassis liqueur

1 tsp sugar or Splenda (no-calorie sweetener)

2 tbsp water

Add onion, celery, salt, and pepper to ground venison. Place 2 bouillon cubes in hot water and add to the venison. Add eggs and cracker meal to the above, mix thoroughly. Form the mixture into a loaf and place in a greased (with olive or canola oil) pan. Apply glaze (see below) to meatloaf with a pastry brush. Preheat oven to 350°F and bake for 1 hour.

To make the red currant glaze, combine the ingredients over low heat.

Deer/Venison Steak Milano

YIELD: 4 to 6 servings

1 cup Burgundy wine

1 clove garlic, minced extra fine

1 small onion, diced fine

$\frac{1}{4}$ tsp oregano

1 Tablespoon Worcestershire sauce

1 tsp salt (Optional)

$\frac{1}{4}$ tsp pepper

2 tsp dry mustard

1 tbsp sugar or Splenda

2 tbsp omega-3 butter/canola butter (Smart Balance)

1 (2 to 2$\frac{1}{2}$ pounds) venison steak

Combine all ingredients, except steak, and heat until butter is melted. Pour sauce over steak and refrigerate several hours, turning meat frequently. Remove steak from sauce and broil for 5 minutes on each side, basting the meat with the sauce.

Elk or Wapiti (Lakota) is considered one of the finest game meats. Generally, the meat is tender, low in fat, and without a gamey flavor. Elk can be used in other the big game recipes shown. The following are especially good for elk.

Elk Shish Kebob

YIELD: **4 servings**

Marinade:

6 oz canola or olive oil

$\frac{1}{4}$ tsp garlic powder

$\frac{1}{4}$ tsp salt

$\frac{1}{4}$ tsp black pepper

$\frac{1}{4}$ tsp paprika

1 oz Cognac

Kebobs:

1 large can mushroom caps (12)

1 large green pepper, cut into 1-inch pieces

12 cherry tomatoes

1 onion, cut into 1-inch pieces

1 (2–3 pound) elk tenderloin, cut into 1-inch pieces

Mix marinade ingredients in a sauce dish. On a skewer, place 1 mushroom cap, a section of green pepper, 1 cherry tomato, a chunk of onion, and 1 cube of tenderloin. Repeat until skewers are full. Place prepared skewers in marinade for 20 minutes. Drain and broil or grill on both sides until the meat reaches the desired degree of doneness.

Prime Rib of Elk, Au Jus

YIELD: 6 to 8 servings

1 (8–9 pound) standing rib of elk

2 cups of olive oil

3 ribs celery

1 onion, cut in quarters

$\frac{1}{2}$ tsp pickling spices

4 cloves garlic, peeled

4 tbsp salt

1 tbsp pepper

3 tsp paprika

$1\frac{1}{2}$ quarts water

6 beef bouillon cubes

4 oz tomato puree

Marinate elk rib roast in olive oil for 12–24 hours. Drain oil from rib roast and place standing rib in roast pan, bone side down. Add celery, onion, pickling spices, and garlic; season with salt and pepper, and dust with paprika. Bake uncovered in 375°F oven until brown (45 minutes). Add water, reduce oven heat to 325°F and bake covered for 10 minutes per pound. Then, remove roast from pan; cut rib bones off or leave them on as desired

Au jus is prepared by straining the residue in the roast pan (this should yield about 1 quart of liquid). Reheat the quart of strained juice, dissolve bouillon cubes into the hot liquid, and add tomato puree. Bring to a boil.

Slice roast into desired number of slices and serve covered with hot au jus.

Low-Carb Grilled Lamb Chops

YIELD: 4 servings

1 tsp ground cumin

1 tsp ground coriander

$\frac{1}{4}$ tsp salt

$\frac{1}{8}$ tsp cinnamon

¹/₈ tsp cayenne pepper

1 tbsp olive or canola oil

4 center cut loin lamb chops, 1-inch thick

2 cloves garlic, minced

Combine cumin, coriander, salt, cinnamon, cayenne pepper, and oil in a small bowl. Rub oil/spice mixture over both sides of lamb chops. Sprinkle garlic over both sides of lamb chops. Grill on medium heat, 4 minutes per side (for medium rare) to 5 minutes (for medium).

Braised Lamb Shanks

YIELD: *4 servings*

2 tbsp whole-wheat flour

1 tsp salt

¹/₂ tsp freshly ground black pepper

4 meaty (l-pound) lamb shanks

3 tbsp olive oil, divided

1 tbsp butter

1 large onion, chopped

4 cloves garlic, minced

1 cup chicken or beef broth

1 cup burgundy or dry red wine

2 tbsp fresh rosemary, chopped (or 2 tsp dried rosemary)

Salt and pepper

Preheat oven to 350°F. Combine flour, salt, and pepper in paper bag. Add shanks one at a time and shake to coat lightly. Heat 2 tablespoons oil and butter in a Dutch oven over medium heat. Add shanks in batches, brown on all sides, then transfer to a plate; set aside.

Add remaining oil to pan, then add onion and garlic and cook for 5 minutes. Add broth, wine, and rosemary, mix, and bring to boil. Return lamb to the pan, cover, and transfer to oven and braise for 1¹/₂ to 2 hours or until tender. Transfer the shanks to a serving platter. Skim off the fat from the pan juices. Boil juices gently until reduced to 2 cups and slightly thickened. Pour sauce over shanks, then season with salt and pepper to taste.

Wild Duck with Rice

YIELD: 4 servings

2 wild ducks, skinned, deboned and cut into $1/2$-inch chunks
$1/4$ cup omega-3 butter/canola butter (Smart Balance)
1 (16-oz) can tomato sauce
4 oz dry white wine
2 cloves garlic, minced very fine
$1/2$ onion, chopped fine
1 rib celery, diced fine
1 medium green pepper, diced medium
Salt and pepper
Dash cayenne pepper (optional)
Wild rice

Sauté the duck in butter in a large frying pan. Add the tomato sauce, wine, garlic, onion, celery, and green pepper. Season to taste with salt, pepper, and cayenne. Heat until boiling. Wild rice should be partially precooked. Add the rice, and stir thoroughly. Simmer over low heat, covered, until the rice is cooked (approximately 20 minutes).

Breast of Pheasant, Partridge, or Quail Cordon Bleu

YIELD: 1 to 2 servings

1 deboned breast (partridge, pheasant, or quail)
Salt and pepper
1 thin slice of smoked ham, per breast
1 slice of Swiss cheese, per breast
1 omega-3 egg white, beaten
Egg wash: 1 omega-3 egg and 1 tbsp skim milk, beaten together
$1/2$ cup of breading (whole wheat or multigrain with seasoned coating mix)

Flatten the breast with a cleaver, then season with salt and pepper. Place ham and cheese into each seasoned breast. Flatten edges to seal ham-and-cheese mixture in the breast. Brush with egg white, and freeze. Dip in egg wash, coat with breading, and refreeze. Fry in a deep-fryer (using canola oil) until golden brown, then bake 45–60 minutes in a 375°F oven.

Pheasant, Quail, or Partridge Cacciatore

YIELD: 4 to 6 servings

3 game birds, cleaned and disjointed

$1/2$ cup whole-wheat flour,
seasoned to taste with salt and pepper

$1/2$ cup canola or cooking oil

1 onion, chopped coarsely

1 green pepper, diced coarsely

2 cloves garlic, diced to a pulp

$1/2$ cup canned mushroom caps

1 can crushed tomatoes with juice

1 cup of Madeira wine

$1/4$ tsp crushed oregano

$1/4$ tsp sweet basil

$1/4$ tsp salt (optional)

$1/4$ tsp black pepper

Dip birds in seasoned flour. Sauté birds in hot cooking oil (canola or olive oil) in a heavy pan until golden brown. Remove and place in a roasting pan or baking dish. Sauté the onion, green pepper, garlic, and mushrooms in a small pan with a little canola oil until golden brown. Add the tomatoes with juice, wine, and seasonings. Mix well and pour over the game birds. Cover and bake at 350°F for approximately 1 hour or until birds are tender.

Breast of Canadian Goose in White Wine Sauce

YIELD: 4 servings

$1/3$ cup whole-wheat flour

$1/2$ tsp salt

$1/4$ tsp pepper

1 breast of goose, skinned and deboned (2 fillets)

$1/4$ cup omega-3 butter/canola butter (Smart Balance)

$1/4$ onion, diced very fine

1 pint Basic Low-Calorie Cream Sauce (see below)

2 oz dry white wine

1 oz brandy or cognac

Mix the whole-wheat flour, salt, and pepper together. Dredge the goose fillets in the seasoned flour. Sauté the floured goose fillets in butter in heavy frying pan until golden brown. Add the diced onion and sauté until translucent. Add the cream sauce, wine, and brandy; salt and pepper to taste. Simmer, covered, for approximately 45 minutes to 1 hour.

Basic Low-Calorie Cream Sauce

YIELD: 8 cups

$1/2$ pound of omega-3 butter/canola butter (Smart Balance)

4 cups whole wheat flour

2 cups water

2 cups skim milk

5 chicken bouillon cubes

Salt and pepper

Heat the butter until it foams, being careful not to scorch it. Slowly add flour, stirring constantly with a wire whisk until the roux mixture loses its sheen and acquires a dull appearance. Remove the butter roux from the heat. Mix milk and water, then heat. Dissolve the bouillon cubes. Season to taste with salt and pepper. Heat to very hot but do not boil. Thicken mixture by adding small amounts of butter roux while stirring continuously with a wire whisk, until it reaches a medium-thick consistency. Remove from heat. (Yellow food coloring may be added).

Wild Turkey with Wild Rice Stuffing

YIELD: *4 to 6 servings*

Basic Stuffing (see below)

2 cups cooked wild rice

*$^3/_4$ cup omega-3 butter/canola butter
(Smart Balance), melted and divided*

1 whole (8–10 pound) wild turkey

$^1/_2$ tsp oregano

$^1/_4$ tsp salt

$^1/_4$ tsp pepper

Mix 3 cups of Basic Stuffing with the wild rice, $^1/_4$ cup melted butter, and $^1/_4$ tsp oregano. Stuff the bird cavity with the mixture. Brush turkey with the mixture of $^1/_2$ cup melted better, $^1/_4$ tsp salt, $^1/_4$ tsp pepper, and $^1/_4$ tsp oregano. Place in baking pan, cover with foil tent, and bake in medium oven (350°F for 15 minutes per pound.) Thirty minutes before removing from oven, remove foil and continue baking until brown. Brush occasionally with seasoned butter mixture.

Basic Stuffing

YIELD: *2$^1/_4$ cups*

$^1/_2$ cup water

$^1/_4$ cup celery, chopped

$^1/_4$ cup onions, chopped

$^1/_4$ cup omega-3 butter

$^1/_8$ tsp poultry seasoning

$^1/_4$ tsp salt

$^1/_4$ tsp sage

1 tsp parsley, chopped

1$^1/_2$ cups of whole-wheat, seasoned bread crumbs

Combine water, celery, and onions and sauté in butter until lightly browned. Add seasonings and bread crumbs, tossing to blend.

Optional ingredients: fresh diced apples, raisins, or other fruit.

Parmesan Turkey Breast

YIELD: 4 servings

$\frac{1}{2}$ tsp salt

$\frac{1}{4}$ tsp freshly ground black pepper

1 pound turkey breast

2 tbsp omega-3 butter/canola butter (Smart Balance), melted

2 cloves garlic, minced

$\frac{1}{2}$ cup grated Parmesan cheese

1 cup spicy marinara sauce

2 tbsp fresh basil or Italian parsley, chopped

Preheat broiler. Sprinkle salt and pepper over turkey. Place turkey in a single layer in a jellyroll pan and brush butter and garlic over turkey. Broil 4 to 5 inches from heat source for 2 minutes and turn. Top with cheese and continue to broil for 2–3 minutes until no longer pink in the middle. Transfer to serving plates; spoon sauce over turkey, and top with basil.

Fillet of Lake Trout with Bercy Butter

YIELD: 4 servings

4 (8-oz) trout fillets

4 tbsp omega-3/canola butter (Smart Balance), melted

Salt and pepper, Paprika

Bercy Butter:

$\frac{1}{2}$ cup omega-3 butter/canola butter (Smart Balance),
at room temperature

2 tbsp white wine

$\frac{1}{2}$ clove garlic, minced extremely fine

1 green onion, diced very fine

Dash cayenne

Brush fillets with melted plain butter. Season with salt and pepper and dust with paprika. Place under broiler, turn once. Cook until meat flakes off with a fork. Remove from heat and top with Bercy Butter (see below).

To form Bercy Butter, mix thoroughly $\frac{1}{2}$ cup of soft butter, white wine, garlic, green onion, and cayenne. Let stand for 15 minutes before using.

Lake Trout Baked with Herbs

YIELD: 1 serving (per fillet)

1 (8-oz) trout fillet per person

4 tbsp omega-3 butter/canola butter (Smart Balance), melted

Salt and pepper

Basil

Thyme

1 lemon, sliced thin

1 orange, sliced thin

Paprika

Place fillets on baking sheet. Brush with melted butter. Season to taste with salt, pepper, basil, and thyme. Alternate lemon and orange slices on top of fillet, then dust with paprika. Bake at 375°F for about 15 minutes.

Grilled Salmon Fillets with Asparagus and Onions

YIELD: 6 servings

$1/3$ tsp paprika

6 salmon fillets (6–8 ounces)

Fresh asparagus spears (1 bunch or pound)

1 red or sweet onion, cut into $1/4$-inch slices

1 tbsp olive oil

Salt and pepper

Marinade:

$1/3$ cup of honey

1 tsp of Dijon mustard

Sprinkle paprika over salmon. Brush marinade over salmon and let stand for 20 minutes. Brush asparagus and onion slices with olive or canola oil and season with salt and pepper to taste (use a salt substitute if you have high blood pressure). Place salmon, skin down, in center of grill over medium coals. Arrange asparagus and onions around salmon and cover grill for 5 minutes, then turn vegetables and salmon and cook another 5–6 minutes or until salmon flakes easily and vegetables are crisp-tender. Separate onion slices into rings and arrange over asparagus.

Raspberry Salsa Walleye

YIELD: 4 servings

4 walleye fillets

1 tbsp olive oil

$\frac{1}{4}$ tsp minced garlic

$\frac{1}{4}$ tsp salt

Raspberry Salsa:

$\frac{3}{4}$ cup fresh raspberry
(consider pineapple as a substitute)

2 tbsp red bell pepper, finely chopped

2 tbsp fresh cilantro, chopped

1 tbsp olive oil

2 tsp minced ginger

1 tsp minced jalapeno pepper

Brush walleye with oil and garlic and sprinkle with salt. Grill walleye, on uncovered grill, over medium-hot coals for 8–10 minutes or until walleye flakes easily. Turn once. Top walleye with salsa and serve.

For the salsa, combine raspberries, bell pepper, cilantro, oil, ginger, and jalapeno pepper into small bowl; mix well. Cover and refrigerate.

APPENDIX B

Food Diary and Weight Loss Record

FOOD DIARY		
Date	Weight	

Time of Day	Food	Calories
		Total

Type of Exercise	Amount

WEIGHT LOSS RECORD	
Month	Weight
1	
2	
3	
4	
5	
6	
7	
8	
9	
10	
11	
12	
13	
14	
15	
16	
17	
18	
19	
20	
21	
22	
23	
24	
25	
26	
27	
28	
29	
30	
31	

References

Health Benefits of Fish

Brown, K.M., and J.R. Arthur. "Selenium, Selnoproteins and Human Health: A Review." *Public Health Nutr* 4:2B (2001): 593–599.

Connor, W. "Will the Dietary Intake of Fish Prevent Atherosclerosis in Diabetic Women?" *Am J Clin Nutr* 80:3 (2004): 535–536.

Erkkila, A., A. Lichtenstein, D. Mozaffarian, and D. Herrington. "Fish Intake is Associated with a Reduced Progression of Coronary Artery Atherosclerosis in Postmenopausal Women with Coronary Artery Disease." *Am J Clin Nutr* 80:3 (2004): 626–632.

Fernandez, E., L. Chatenoud, C. La Vecchia, et al. "Fish Consumption and Cancer Risk." *Am J Clin Nutr* 70:1 (1999): 85–90.

He, K., Y. Song, M.L. Daviglus, et al. "Fish Consumption and Incidence of Stroke: A Meta-analysis of Cohort Studies." *Stroke* 35:7 (2004): 1538–1542.

Iso, H., K.M. Rexrode, M.J. Stampfer, et al. "Intake of Fish and Omega-3 Fatty Acids and Risk of Stroke in Women." *JAMA* 285:3 (2001): 304–312.

Kalmijn, S., M.P. van Boxtel, M. Ocke, et al. "Dietary Intake of Fatty Acids and Fish in Relation to Cognitive Performance at Middle Age." *Neurology* 62:2 (2004): 275–280.

Morris, M.C., D.A. Evans, J.L. Bienias, et al. "Consumption of Fish and n-3 Fatty Acids and Risk of Incident Alzheimer Disease." *Arch Neurol* 60:7 (2003): 940–946.

Petrik, M.B., M.F. McEntee, B.T. Johnson, et al. "Highly Unsaturated (n-3) Fatty Acids, but Not Alpha-linolenic, Conjugated Linoleic or Gamma-linolenic Acids, Reduce Tumorigenesis in Apc(Min/+) Mice." *J Nutr* 130:10 (2000): 2434–2443.

Phelan, S., J.O. Hill, W. Lang, et al. "Recovery from Relapse Among Successful Weight Maintainers." *Am J Clin Nutr* 78 (2003): 1079–1084.

Serhan, C.N., S. Hong, K. Gronert, et al. "Resolvins: A Family of Bioactive Products of Omega-3 Fatty Acid Transformation Circuits Initiated by Aspirin Treatment that Counter Proinflammation Signals." *J Exp Med* 196:8 (2002): 1025–1037.

Vogt, T.M., R.G. Ziegler, B.I. Graubard, et al. "Serum Selenium and Risk of Prostate Cancer in U.S. Blacks and Whites." *Int J Cancer* 103:5 (2003): 664–670.

Foods From Grass-Fed Animals

Aro, A., S. Mannisto, I. Salminen, et al. "Inverse Association Between Dietary and Serum Conjugated Linoleic Acid and Risk of Breast Cancer in Postmenopausal Women." *Nutr Cancer* 38:2 (2000): 151–157.

Chin, S.F., et al. "Dietary Sources of Conjugated Dienoic Isomers of Linoleic Acid, a Newly Recognized Class of Anticarcinogens." *J Food Composition* 5 (1992): 185–197.

Cordain, L., et al. "A Detailed Fatty Acid Analysis of Selected Tissues in Elk, Mule Deer, and Antelope." *Food Composition* 670.1–670.6.

Davidson, M.H., D. Hunninghake, et al. "Comparison of the Effects of Lean Red Meat vs. Lean White Meat on Serum Lipid Levels Among Free-living Persons with Hypercholesterolemia: A Long-term, Randomized Clinical Trial." *Arch Intern Med* 159:12 (1999): 1331–1338.

Duckett, S.K., D.G. Wagner, et al. "Effects of Time on Feed on Beef Nutrient Composition." *J Anim Sci* 71:8 (1993): 2079–2088.

Ip, C., J.A. Scimeca, et al. "Conjugated Linoleic Acid: A Powerful Anti-carcinogen From Animal Fat Sources." *Cancer* 74:3 Suppl (1994): 1050–1054.

Langlois, B.E., K.A. Dawson, et al. "Effect of Age and Housing Location on Antibiotic Resistance of Fecal Coliforms From Pigs in a Non-antibiotic-exposed Herd." *Appl Environ Microbiol* 54:6 (1988): 1341–1344.

Lopez-Bote, C.J., R. Sanz Arias, A.I. Rey, et al. "Effect of Free-range Feeding on Omega-3 Fatty Acids and Alpha-tocopherol Content and Oxidative Stability of Eggs." *Animal Feed Sci Technol* 72 (1998): 33–40.

Rose, D.P., J.M. Connolly, et al. "Influence of Diets Containing Eicosapentaenoic or Docasahexaenoic Acid on Growth and Metastasis of Breast Cancer Cells in Nude Mice." *J Natl Cancer Inst* 87:8 (1995): 587–592.

Rule, D.C., K.S. Broughton, S.M. Shellito, and G. Maiorano. "Comparison of Muscle Fatty Acid Profiles and Cholesterol Concentrations of Bison, Beef Cattle, Elk, and Chicken." *J Anim Sci* 80:5 (2002): 1202–1211.

Russell, J.B., F. Diez-Gonzalez, and G.N. Jarvis. "Potential Effect of Cattle Diets on the Transmission of Pathogenic Escherichia Coli to Humans." *Microbes Infect* 2:1 (2000): 45–53.

Shaver, Randy D. "By-Product Feedstuffs in Dairy Cattle Diets in the Upper Midwest." Department of Dairy Science, College of Agricultural and Life Sciences, University of Wisconsin.

Simopolous, A.P., and J. Robinson. *The Omega Diet.* New York: HarperCollins, 1999.

Siscovick, D.S., T.E. Raghunathan, et al. "Dietary Intake and Cell Membrane Levels of Long-Chain n-3 Polyunsaturated Fatty Acids and the Risk of Primary Cardiac Arrest." *JAMA* 274:17 (1995): 1363–1367.

Smith, G.C. "Dietary Supplementation of Vitamin E to Cattle to Improve Shelf Life and

Case Life of Beef for Domestic and International Markets." Colorado State University, Fort Collins, Colorado.

Stockdale, C.R., G.P. Walker, et al. "Influence of Pasture and Concentrates in the Diet of Grazing Dairy Cows on the Fatty Acid Composition of Milk." *J Dairy Res* 70:3 (2003): 267–276.

Tashiro, T., H. Yamamori, et al. "N-3 versus n-6 Polyunsaturated Fatty Acids in Critical Illness." *Nutrition* 14:6 (1998): 551–553.

Tisdale, M.J. "Wasting in Cancer." *J Nutr* 129:1 Suppl (1995): 243S–246S.

Homocysteine and Heart Disease

Bazzano, L.A., J. He, L.G. Odgen, et al. "Dietary Intake of Folate and Risk of Stroke in U.S. Men and Women: NHANES I Epidemiologic Follow-up Study." *Stroke* 33:5 (2002): 1183–1189.

Berg, M.J. "The Importance of Folic Acid." *J Gend Specif Med* 2:3 (1999): 24–28.

Clarke, R., et al. "Hyperhomocystenemia: An Independent Risk Factor for Heart Disease." *New Engl J Med* 324 (1991): 1149–1155.

De Vriese, A.S., J.H. De Sutter, et al. "Mild to Moderate Hyperhomocystenemia in Cardiovascular Disease." *Acta Cardiol* 53:6 (1998): 337–344.

Glueck, C.J., et al. "Evidence That Homocysteine is an Independent Risk Factor." *Am J Cardiol* (1995): 132–136.

Flaxseed and Health

Allman, M.A., M.M. Pena, and D. Pang. "Supplementation with Flaxseed Oil versus Sunflower Seed Oil in Healthy Young Men Consuming a Low Fat Diet: Effects on Platelet Composition and Function." *Eur J Clin Nutr* 49:3 (1995): 169–178.

Bazzano, L.A., J. He, L.G. Ogden, et al. "Dietary Fiber Intake and Reduced Risk of Coronary Heart Disease in U.S. Men and Women: The National Health and Nutrition Examination Survey I Epidemiologic Follow-up Study." *Arch Intern Med* 163:16 (2003): 1897–1904.

Carter, J.P., et al. "Hypothesis: Dietary Management May Improve Survival from Nutritionally Linked Cancers Based on Analysis of Representative Cases." *J Am College Nutr* 12 (1993): 209–226.

Chung, T.W., J.J. Yu, and D.Z. Liu. "Reducing Lipid Peroxidation Stress of Erythrocyte Membrane by Alpha-tocopherol Nicotinate Plays an Important Role in Improving Blood Rheological Properties in Type 2 Diabetic Patients with Retinopathy." *Diabet Med* 15:5 (1998): 380–385.

Cleland, L.G., and M.J. James. "Rheumatoid Arthritis and the Balance of Dietary n-6 and n-3 Essential Fatty Acids." *Br J Rheumatol* 36:5 (1997): 513–514.

Colditz, G.A., J.E. Manson, et al. "Diet and Risk of Clinical Diabetes in Women." *Am J Clin Nutr* 55:5 (1992): 1018–1023.

Cunnane, S.C., M.J. Hamadeh, A.C. Liede, et al. "Nutritional Attributes of Traditional Flaxseed in Healthy Young Adults." *Am J Clin Nutr* 61:1 (1995): 62–68.

Darlington, G., A. Jump, and N. Ramsey. "Dietary Treatment of Rheumatoid Arthritis." *Practitioner* 234:1488 (1990): 456–460.

Kurzer, M.S., J.W. Lampe, M.C. Martini, et al. "Fecal Lignan and Isoflavonoid Excretion in Premenopausal Women Consuming Flaxseed Powder." *Cancer Epidemiol Biomarkers Prev* 4:4 (1995): 353–358.

Mantzioris, E., M.J. James, R.A. Gibson, et al. "Nutritional Attributes of Dietary Flaxseed Oil." *Am J Clin Nutr* 62:4 (1995): 841–842.

Nesbitt, P.D., and L.U. Thompson. "Lignans in Homemade and Commercial Products Containing Flaxseed." *Nutr Cancer* 29:3 (1997): 222–227.

Health Benefits of Walnuts

Fukuda, T., H. Ito, and T. Yoshida. "Antioxidative Polyphenols from Walnuts." *Phytochemistry* 63:7 (YEAR?): 795–801.

Morgan, J.M., K. Horton, D. Reese, et al. "Effects of Walnut Consumption as Part of a Low-fat, Low-cholesterol Diet on Serum Cardiovascular Risk Factors." *Int J Vitam Nutr Res* 72:5 (2002): 341–347.

Ros, E., I. Nunez, A. Perez-Heras, et al. "A Walnut Diet Improves Endothelial Function in Hypercholesterolemic Subjects: A Randomized Crossover Trial." *Circulation* 109:13 (2004): 1609–1614.

Stevens, L.J., S.S. Zentall, M.L. Abate, et al. "Omega-3 Fatty Acids in Boys with Behavior, Learning, and Health Problems." *Physiol Behav* 59:4/5 (1996): 915–920.

Stevens, L.J., S.S. Zentall, J.L. Deck, et al. "Essential Fatty Acid Metabolism in Boys with Attention-Deficit Hyperactivity Disorder." *Am J Clin Nutr* 62:4 (1995): 761–768.

Tapsell, L.C., L.J. Gillen, C.S. Patch, et al. "Including Walnuts in a Low-Fat/Modified-Fat Diet Improves HDL Cholesterol-to-Total Cholesterol Ratios in Patients With Type 2 Diabetes." *Diabetes Care* 27:12 (2004): 2777–2783.

Fruits of the Dakotas

Bazzano, L.A., J. He, L.G. Ogden, et al. "Dietary Fiber Intake and Reduced Risk of Coronary Heart Disease in U.S. Men and Women: The National Health and Nutrition Examination Survey I Epidemiologic Follow-up Study." *Arch Intern Med* 163:16 (2003): 1897–1904.

Boyer, J., and R.H. Liu. "Apple Phytochemicals and Their Health Benefits." *Nutr J* 3:1 (2004): 5.

Cho, E., J.M. Seddon, B. Rosner, et al. "Prospective Study of Intake of Fruits, Vegetables, Vitamins, and Carotenoids and Risk of Age-related Maculopathy." *Arch Ophthalmol* 122:6 (2004): 883–892.

Edwards, A.J., B.T. Vinyard, E.R. Wiley, et al. "Consumption of Watermelon Juice Increases Plasma Concentrations of Lycopene and Beta-carotene in Humans." *J Nutr* 133:4 (2003): 1043–1050.

Freedman, J.E., C. Parker 3rd, L. Li, et al. "Select Flavonoids and Whole Juice from Purple Grapes Inhibit Platelet Function and Enhance Nitric Oxide Release." *Circulation* 103:23 (2001): 2792–2798.

Hankinson, S.E., M.J Stampfer, J.M. Seddon, et al. "Nutrient Intake and Cataract Extraction in Women: A Prospective Study." *BMJ* 305:6849 (1992): 335–339.

Huxley, R.R., and H.A.W. Neil. "The Relation Between Dietary Flavonol Intake and Coronary Heart Disease Mortality: A Meta-analysis of Prospective Cohort Studies." *Eur J Clin Nutr* 57 (2003): 904–908.

Khaw, K.T., S. Bingham, A. Welch, et al. "Relation Between Plasma Ascorbic Acid and Mortality in Men and Women in EPIC-Norfolk Prospective Study: A Prospective Population Study. European Prospective Investigation into Cancer and Nutrition." *Lancet* 357:9257 (2001): 657–663.

Knekt, P., R. Jarvinen, A. Reunanen, et al. "Flavonoid Intake and Coronary Mortality in Finland: A Cohort Study." *BMJ* 312:7029 (1996): 478–481.

Miyagi, Y., K. Miwa, and H. Inoue. "Inhibition of Human Low-density Lipoprotein Oxidation by Flavonoids in Red Wine and Grape Juice." *Am J Cardiol* 80:12 (1997): 1627–1631.

Pearson, D.A., C.H. Tan, J.B. German, et al. "Apple Juice Inhibits Low-density Lipoprotein Oxidation." *Life Sci* 64:21 (1999): 1913–1920.

Sable-Amplis, R., R. Sicart, R. Agid. "Further Studies on the Cholesterol-lowering Effect of Apple in Humans: Biochemical Mechanisms Involved." *Nutr Res* 3 (1983): 325–328.

Stewart, J.R., M.C. Artime, C.A. O'Brian. "Resveratrol: A Candidate Nutritional Substance for Prostate Cancer Prevention." *J Nutr* 133:7 Suppl (2003): 2440S–2443S.

Vegetables of the Dakotas

Appel, L.J., T.J. Moore, E. Obarzanek, et al. "A Clinical Trial of the Effects of Dietary Patterns on Blood Pressure. DASH Collaborative Research Group." *New Engl J Med* 336:16 (1997): 1117–1124.

Bazzano, L.A., J. He, L.G. Ogden, et al. "Dietary Fiber Intake and Reduced Risk of Coronary Heart Disease in U.S. Men and Women: The National Health and Nutrition Examination Survey I Epidemiologic Follow-up Study." *Arch Intern Med* 163:16 (2003): 1897–1904.

Elkayam, A., D. Mirelman, E. Peleg, et al. "The Effects of Allicin on Weight in Fructose-induced Hyperinsulinemic, Hyperlipidemic, Hypertensive Rats." *Am J Hypertens* 16:12 (2003): 1053–1056.

Erhardt, J.G., C. Meisner, J.C. Bode, et al. "Lycopene, Beta-carotene, and Colorectal Adenomas." *Am J Clin Nutr* 78:6 (2003): 1219–1224.

Fahey, J.W., Y. Zhang, P. Talalay. "Broccoli Sprouts: An Exceptionally Rich Source of Inducers of Enzymes that Protect Against Chemical Carcinogens." *Proc Natl Acad Sci* 94 (1997): 10367–10372.

Grube, B.J., E.T. Eng, Y.C. Kao, et al. "White Button Mushroom Phytochemicals Inhibit Aromatase Activity and Breast Cancer Cell Proliferation." *J Nutr* 131:12 (2001): 3288–3293.

Holguin, F., M.M. Tellez-Rojo, M. Lazo, et al. "Cardiac Autonomic Changes Associated with Fish Oil vs Soy Oil Supplementation in the Elderly." *Chest* 127:4 (2005): 1102–1107.

Huxley, R.R., and H.A.W. Neil. "The Relation Between Dietary Flavonol Intake and Coronary Heart Disease Mortality: A Meta-analysis of Prospective Cohort Studies." *Eur J Clin Nutr* 57 (2003): 904–908.

Joseph, J.A., B. Shukitt-Hale, N.A. Denisova, et al. "Long-term Dietary Strawberry, Spinach or Vitamin E Supplementation Retards the Onset of Age-related Neuronal Signal-transduction and Cognitive Behavioral Deficits." *J Neurosci* 18:19 (1998): 8047–8055.

Joseph, J.A., B. Shukitt-Hale, N.A. Denisova, et al. "Reversals of Age-related Declines in Neuronal Signal Transduction, Cognitive, and Motor Behavioral Deficits with Blueberry, Spinach, or Strawberry Dietary Supplementation." *J Neurosci* 19:18 (1999): 8114–8121.

Khaw, K.T., S. Bingham, A. Welch, et al. "Relation Between Plasma Ascorbic Acid and Mortality in Men and Women in EPIC-Norfolk Prospective Study: A Prospective Population Study. European Prospective Investigation into Cancer and Nutrition." *Lancet* 357:9257 (2001): 657–663.

Kritz-Silverstein, D., and D.L. Goodman-Gruen. "Usual Dietary Isoflavone Intake, Bone Mineral Density, and Bone Metabolism in Postmenopausal Women." *J Women's Health Gend Based Med* 11:1 (2002): 69–78.

Kusano, S., and H. Abe. "Antidiabetic Activity of White Skinned Sweet Potato in Obese Zucker Fatty Rats". *Biol Pharm Bull* 23:1 (2000): 23–26.

Lee, M.M., S.L. Gomez, J.S. Chang, et al. "Soy and Isoflavone Consumption in Relation to Prostate Cancer Risk in China." *Cancer Epidemiol Biomarkers* 12:7 (2003): 665–668.

Levy, J. Lycopene research presented at the annual meeting of the American Association for Cancer Research, March 27–31, 2004, Orlando, Florida.

Longnecker, M.P., P.A. Newcomb, R. Mittendorf, et al. "Intake of Carrots, Spinach, and Supplements Containing Vitamin A in Relation to Risk of Breast Cancer." *Cancer Epidemiol Biomarkers Prev* 6:11 (1997): 887–892.

Lu, Q.Y., J.C. Hung, D. Heber, et al. "Inverse Associations Between Plasma Lycopene and Other Carotenoids and Prostate Cancer." *Cancer Epidemiol Biomarkers Prev* 10:7 (2001): 749–756.

Morris, M.C., D.A. Evans, J.L. Bienias, et al. "Dietary Niacin and the Risk of Incident Alzheimer's Disease and of Cognitive Decline." *J Neurol Neurosurg Psychiatry* 75:8 (2004): 1093–1099.

Pattison, D.J., A.J. Silman, N.J. Goodson, et al. "Vitamin C and the Risk of Developing Inflammatory Polyarthritis: Prospective Nested Case-control Study." *Ann Rheum Dis* 63:7 (2004): 843–847.

Reboul, E., P. Borel, C. Mikail, et al. "Enrichment of Tomato Paste with 6% Tomato Peel Increases Lycopene and Beta-carotene Bioavailability in Men." *J Nutr* 135:4 (2005): 790–794.

Richardson, K. "Soy Could Be Good for the Heart and Bones of Premenopausal Women."

Research conducted at Wake Forest University Baptist Medical Center and presented at the annual meeting of the North American Menopause Society, October 6–9, 2004, Washington, D.C.

Sueda, S., H. Fukuda, K. Watanabe, et al. "Magnesium Deficiency in Patients with Recent Myocardial Infarction and Provoked Coronary Artery Spasm." *Jpn Circ J* 65:7 (2001): 643–648.

Tavani, A., E. Negri, C. La Vecchia. "Food and Nutrient Intake and Risk of Cataract." *Ann Epidemiol* 6:1 (1996): 41–46.

Wagner, J.D., D.C. Schwenke, K.A. Greaves, et al. "Soy Protein with Isoflavones, but Not an Isoflavone-rich Supplement, Improves Arterial Low-density Lipoprotein Metabolism and Atherogenesis." *Arterioscler Thromb Vasc Biol* 23:12 (2003): 2241–2246.

Wilt, T.J., A. Ishani, I. Rutks, et al. "Phytotherapy for Benign Prostatic Hyperplasia." *Public Health Nutr* 3:4A (2000): 459–472.

Wood, C.E., T.C. Register, M.S. Anthony, et al. "Breast and Uterine Effects of Soy Isoflavones and Conjugated Equine Estrogens in Postmenopausal Female Monkeys." *J Clin Endocrinol Metab* 89:7 (2004): 3462–3468.

Wu, L., M.H. Ashraf, M. Facci, et al. "Dietary Approach to Attenuate Oxidative Stress, Hypertension, and Inflammation in the Cardiovascular System." *Proc Natl Acad Sci USA* 101:18 (2004): 7094–7099.

Yamamoto, S., T. Sobue, M. Kobayashi, et al. "Soy, Isoflavones, and Breast Cancer Risk in Japan." *J Natl Cancer Inst* 95:12 (2003): 906–913.

Yamamoto, J., T. Taka, K. Yamada, et al. "Tomatoes have Natural Anti-thrombotic Effects." *Br J Nutr* 90:6 (2003): 1031–1038.

Zhan, S., and S.C. Ho. "Meta-analysis of the Effects of Soy Protein Containing Isoflavones on the Lipid Profile." *Am J Clin Nutr* 81:2 (2005): 397–408.

Zhang, J., J.C. Hsu, M.A. Kinseth, et al. "Indole-3-carbinol Induces a G1 Cell Cycle Arrest and Inhibits Prostate-specific Antigen Production in Human *LNCaP* Prostate Carcinoma Cells." *Cancer* 98:11 (2003): 2511–2520.

Grains, Fiber, and Health

Anderson, J.W., T.J. Hanna, X. Peng, et al. "Whole-grain Foods and Heart Disease Risk." J *Am Coll Nutr* 19:3 Suppl (2000): 291S–299S.

Bansal, H.C., K.N. Strivastava, B.O. Eggum, et al. "Nutritional Evaluation of High-protein Genotypes of Barley." *J Sci Food Agric* 28:2 (1977): 157–160.

Bazzano, L.A., J. He, L.G. Ogden, et al. "Dietary Fiber Intake and Reduced Risk of Coronary Heart Disease in U.S. Men and Women: The National Health and Nutrition Examination Survey I Epidemiologic Follow-up Study." *Arch Intern Med* 163:16 (2003): 1897–1904.

Behall, K.M., D.J. Scholfield, J. Hallfrisch. "Diets Containing Barley Significantly Reduce Lipids in Mildly Hypercholesterolemic Men and Women." *Am J Clin Nutr* 80:5 (2004): 1185–1193.

Craig, W. "Phytochemicals: Guardians of Our Health." *J Am Diet Assoc* 97:Suppl 2 (1997): S199–S204.

Gabrovska, D., V. Fiedlerova, M. Holasova, et al. "The Nutritional Evaluation of Underutilized Cereals and Buckwheat." *Food Nutr Bull* 23:3 Suppl (2002): 246–249.

He, J., M.J. Klag, P.K. Whelton, et al. "Oats and Buckwheat Intakes and Cardiovascular Disease Risk Factors in an Ethnic Minority of China." *Am J Clin Nutr* 61:2 (1995): 366–372.

Jacobs, D.R., M.A. Pereira, K.A. Meyer, et al. "Fiber from Whole Grains, but Not Refined Grains, is Inversely Associated with All-cause Mortality in Older Women: The Iowa Women's Health Study." *J Am Coll Nutr* 19:3 Suppl (2000): 326S–330S.

Jensen, M.K., P. Koh-Banerjee, F.B. Hu, et al. "Intakes of Whole Grains, Bran, and Germ and the Risk of Coronary Heart Disease in Men." *Am J Clin Nutr* 80:6 (2004): 1492–1499.

Liu, L., L. Zubik, F.W. Collins, et al. "The Antiatherogenic Potential of Oat Phenolic Compounds." *Atherosclerosis* 175:1 (2004): 39–49.

Liu, R.H. "New Finding May Be Key to Ending Confusion Over Link Between Fiber, Colon Cancer." American Institute for Cancer Research Press Release, November 3, 2004.

Liu, S., W.C. Willett, J.E. Manson, et al. "Relation Between Changes in Intakes of Dietary Fiber and Grain Products and Changes in Weight and Development of Obesity Among Middle-aged Women." *Am J Clin Nutr* 78:5 (2003): 920–927.

McKeown, N.M., J.B. Meigs, S. Liu, et al. "Carbohydrate Nutrition, Insulin Resistance, and the Prevalence of the Metabolic Syndrome in the Framingham Offspring Cohort." *Diabetes Care* 27:2 (2004): 538–546.

Middleton, E., and C. Kandaswami. "Effects of Flavonoids on Immune and Inflammatory Cell Functions." *Biochem Pharmacol* 43:6 (1992): 1167–1179.

Omega-3 Fatty Acids

Albert, C.M., C.H. Hennekens, C.J. O'Donnell, et al. "Fish Consumption and Risk of Sudden Cardiac Death." *JAMA* 279:1 (1998): 23–28.

Ando, H., A. Ryu, A. Hashimoto, et al. "Linoleic Acid and Alpha-linolenic Acid Lightens Ultraviolet-induced Hyperpigmentation of the Skin." *Arch Dermatol Res* 290:7 (1998): 375–381.

Appel, L.J. "Nonpharmacologic Therapies that Reduce Blood Pressure: A Fresh Perspective." *Clin Cardiol* 22:Suppl III (1999): III1–III5.

Arnold, L.E., D. Kleykamp, N. Votolato, et al. "Potential Link Between Dietary Intake of Fatty Acid and Behavior: Pilot Exploration of Serum Lipids in Attention-deficit Hyperactivity Disorder." *J Child Adolesc Psychopharmacol* 4:3 (1994): 171–182.

Aronson, W.J., J.A. Glaspy, S.T. Reddy, et al. "Modulation of Omega-3/Omega-6 Polyunsaturated Ratios with Dietary Fish Oils in Men with Prostate Cancer." *Urology* 58:2 (2001): 283–288.

Baumgaertel, A. "Alternative and Controversial Treatments for Attention-deficit/hyperactivity Disorder." *Pediatr Clin North Am* 46:5 (1999): 977–992.

Belluzzi, A., S. Boschi, C. Brignola, et al. "Polyunsaturated Fatty acids and Inflammatory Bowel Disease." *Am J Clin Nutr* 71:Suppl (2000): 339S–342S.

Belluzzi, A., C. Brignolia, M. Campieri, et al. "Effect of an Enteric-coated Fish-oil Preparation on Relapses in Crohn's Disease." *New Engl J Med* 334:24 (1996): 1558–1560.

Brown, D.J., and A.M. Dattner. "Phytotherapeutic Approaches to Common Dermatologic Conditions." *Arch Dermtol* 134 (1998): 1401–1404.

Burgess, J., L. Stevens, W. Zhang, et al. "Long-chain Polyunsaturated Fatty Acids in Children with Attention-deficit Hyperactivity Disorder." *Am J Clin Nutr* 71:Suppl (2000): 327S–330S.

Calder, P.C. "N-3 Polyunsaturated Fatty Acids, Inflammation and Immunity: Pouring Oil on Troubled Waters or Another Fishy Tale?" *Nutr Res* 21 (2001): 309–341.

Cho, E., S. Hung, W.C. Willet, et al. "Prospective Study of Dietary Fat and the Risk of Age-related Macular Degeneration." *Am J Clin Nutr* 73:2 (2001): 209–218.

Christensen, J.H., H.A. Skou, L. Fog, et al. "Marine n-3 Fatty Acids, Wine Intake, and Heart Rate Variability in Patients Referred for Coronary Angiography." *Circulation* 103 (2001): 623–625.

Connor, S.L., and W.E. Connor. "Are fish oils beneficial in the prevention and treatment of coronary artery disease?" *Am J Clin Nutr* 66:Suppl (1997): 1020S–1031S.

Curtis, C..L, C.E. Hughes, C.R. Flannery, et al. "N-3 Fatty Acids Specifically Modulate Catabolic Factors Involved in Articular Cartilage Degradation." *J Biol Chem* 275:2 (2000): 721–724.

de Logeril, M., P. Salen, J.L. Martin, et al. "Mediterranean Diet, Traditional Risk Factors, and the Rate of Cardiovascular Complications After Myocardial Infarction: Final Report of the Lyon Diet Heart Study." *Circulation* 99:6 (1999): 779–785.

Deutch, B. "Menstrual Pain in Danish Women Correlated with Low n-3 Polyunsaturated Fatty Acid Intake." *Eur J Clin Nutr* 49:7 (1995): 508–516.

Dewailly, E., C. Blanchet, S. Lemieux, et al. "N-3 Fatty Acids and Cardiovascular Disease Risk Factors Among the Inuit of Nunavik." *Am J Clin Nutr* 74:4 (2001): 464–473.

Dichi, I., P. Frenhane, J.B. Dichi, et al. "Comparison of Omega-3 Fatty Acids and Sulfasalazine in Ulcerative Colitis." *Nutrition* 16 (2000): 87–90.

Edwards, R., M. Peet, J. Shay, et al. "Omega-3 Polyunsaturated Fatty Acid Levels in the Diet and in Red Blood Cell Membranes of Depressed Patients." *J Affect Disord* 48:2–3 (1998): 149–155.

Foulon, T., M.J. Richard, N. Payen, et al. "Effects of Fish Oil Fatty Acids on Plasma Lipids and Lipoproteins and Oxidant-Antioxidant Imbalance in Healthy Subjects." *Scan J Clin Lab Invest* 59:4 (1999): 239–248.

Freeman, V.L., M. Meydan, S. YonG, et al. "Prostatic Levels of Fatty Acids and the Histopathology of Localized Prostate Cancer." *J Urol* 164:6 (2000): 2168–2172.

Friedberg, C.E., M.J. Janssen, R.J. Heine, et al. "Fish Oil and Glycemic Control in Diabetes: A Meta-analysis." *Diabetes Care* 21 (1998): 494–500.

Geerling, B.J., A.C. Houwelingen, A. Badart-Smook, et al. "Fat Intake and Fatty Acid Profile in Plasma Phospholipids and Adipose Tissue in Patients with Crohn's Disease, Compared with Controls." *Am J Gastroenterol* 94:2 (1999): 410–417.

Harbi, M.M., M.W. Islam, O.A. Al-Shabanah, et al. "Effect of Acute Administration of Fish Oil (Omega-3 Marine Triglyceride) on Gastric Ulceration and Secretion Induced by Various Ulcerogenic and Necrotizing Agents in Rats." *Fed Chem Toxic* 33:7 (1995): 555–558.

Harper, C.R., and T.A. Jacobson. "The Fats of Life: The Role of Omega-3 Fatty Acids in the Prevention of Coronary Heart Disease." *Arch Intern Med* 161:18 (2001): 2185–2192.

Hibbeln, J.R. "Fish Consumption and Major Depression." *Lancet* 351:9110 (1998): 1213.

Horrobin, D.F., and C.N. Bennett. "Depression and Bipolar Disorder: Relationships to Impaired Fatty Acid and Phospholipid Metabolism and to Diabetes, Cardiovascular Disease, Immunological Abnormalities, Cancer, Ageing and Osteoporosis." *Prostaglandins Leukot Essent Fatty Acids* 60:4 (1999): 217–234.

Hu, F.B., M.J. Stampfer, J.E. Manson, et al. "Dietary Intake of Alpha-linolenic Acid and Risk of Fatal Ischemic Heart Disease Among Women." *Am J Clin Nutr* 69 (1999): 890–897.

Iso, H., K.M. Rexrode, M.J. Stampfer, et al. "Intake of Fish and Omega-3 Fatty Acids and Risk of Stroke in Women." *JAMA* 285:3 (2001): 304–312.

Juhl, A., J. Marniemi, R. Huupponen, et al. "Effects of Diet and Simvistatin on Serum Lipids, Insulin, and Antioxidants in Hypercholesterolemic Men: A Randomized Controlled Trial." *JAMA* 287:5 (2002): 598–605.

Kremer, J.M. "N-3 Fatty Acid Supplements in Rheumatoid Arthritis." *Am J Clin Nutr* Suppl 1 (2000): 349S–351S.

Kris-Etherton, P., R.H. Eckel, B.V. Howard, et al. "AHA Science Advisory: Lyon Diet Heart Study. Benefits of a Mediterranean-style, National Cholesterol Education Program/American Heart Association Step I Dietary Pattern on Cardiovascular Disease." *Circulation* 103 (2001): 1823.

Kruger, M.C., and D.F. Horrobin. "Calcium Metabolism, Osteoporosis and Essential Fatty Acids: A Review." *Prog Lipid Res* 36 (1997): 131–151.

Laugharne, J.D., J.E. Mellor, M. Peet. "Fatty acids and Schizophrenia." *Lipids* 31:Suppl (1996): S163–S165.

Lockwood, K., S. Moesgaard, T. Hanioka, et al. "Apparent Partial Remission of Breast Cancer in 'High Risk' Patients Supplemented with Nutritional Antioxidants, Essential Fatty Acids, and Coenzyme Q10." *Mol Aspects Med* 15:Suppl (1994): s231–s240.

Lopez-Miranda, J., P. Gomez, P. Castro, et al. "Mediterranean Diet Improves Low-density

Lipoproteins' Susceptibility to Oxidative Modifications." *Med Clin (Barc)* 115:10 (2000): 361–365.

Mayser, P., U. Mrowietz, P. Arenberger, et al. "Omega-3 Fatty Acid–based Lipid Infusion in Patients with Chronic Plaque Psoriasis: Results of a Double-blind, Randomized, Placebo-controlled, Multicenter Trial." *J Am Acad Dermatol* 38:4 (1998): 539–547.

Meydani, M. "Omega-3 Fatty Acids Alter Soluble Markers of Endothelial Function in Coronary Heart Disease Patients." *Nutr Rev* 58:2 Part 1 (2000): 56–59.

Mitchell, E.A., M.G. Aman, S.H. Turbott, et al. "Clinical characteristics and serum essential fatty acid levels in hyperactive children." *Clin Pediatr (Phila)* 26 (1987): 406–411.

Morris, M.C., F. Sacks, B. Rosner. "Does Fish Oil Lower Blood Pressure? A Meta-analysis of Controlled Trials." *Circulation* 88 (1993): 523–533.

Nestel, P.J., S.E. Pomeroy, T. Sasahara, et al. "Arterial Compliance in Obese Subjects is Improved with Dietary Plant n-3 Fatty Acid from Flaxseed Oil Despite Increased LDL Oxidizability." *Arterioscler Thromb Vasc Biol* 17:6 (1997): 1163–1170.

Newcomer, L.M., I.B. King , K.G. Wicklund, et al. "The Association of Fatty Acids with Prostate Cancer Risk." *Prostate* 47:4 (2001): 262–268.

Okamoto, M., F. Misunobu, K. Ashida, et al. "Effects of Dietary Supplementation with n-3 Fatty Acids Compared with n-6 Fatty Acids on Bronchial Asthma." *Intern Med* 39:2 (2000): 107–111.

Olsen, S.F., and N.J. Secher. "Low Consumption of Seafood in Early Pregnancy as a Risk Factor for Preterm Delivery: Prospective Cohort Study." *BMJ* 324:7335 (2002): 447–451.

Prisco, D., R. Paniccia, B. Bandinelli, et al. "Effect of Medium Term Supplementation with a Moderate Dose of n-3 Polyunsaturated Fatty Acid on Blood Pressure in Mild Hypertensive Patients." *Thromb Res* 91 (1998): 105–112.

Richardson, A.J., and B.K. Puri. "The Potential Role of Fatty Acids in Attention-deficit/hyperactivity Disorder." *Prostaglandins Leukot Essent Fatty Acids* 63:1/2 (2000): 79–87.

Sanders, T.A., and A. Hinds. "The Influence of a Fish Oil High in Docosahexaenoic Acid on Plasma Lipoprotein and Vitamin E Concentrations and Haemostatic Function in Healthy Male Volunteers." *Br J Nutr* 68:1 (1992): 163–173.

Simopoulos, A.P. "Essential Fatty Acids in Health and Chronic Disease." *Am J Clin Nutr* 70:30 Suppl (1999): 560S–569S.

Smith, W., P. Mitchell, S.R. Leeder. "Dietary Fat and Fish Intake and Age-related Maculopathy." *Arch Opthamol* 118:3 (2000): 401–404.

Soyland, E., J. Funk, G. Rajka, et al. "Effect of Dietary Supplementation with Very-long Chain n-3 Fatty Acids in Patients with Psoriasis." *N Engl J Med* 328:25 (1993): 1812–1816.

Stark, K.D., E.J. Park, V.A. Maines, et al. "Effect of Fish-oil Concentrate on Serum Lipids in Postmenopausal Women Receiving and Not Receiving Hormone Replacement Therapy in a Placebo-controlled, Double-blind Trial." *Am J Clin Nutr* 72 (2000): 389–394.

Stevens, L.J., S.S. Zentall, M.L. Abate, et al. "Omega-3 Fatty Acids in Boys with Behavior, Learning and Health Problems." *Physiol Behav* 59:4/5 (1996): 915–920.

Stoll, B.A. "Breast Cancer and the Western Diet: Role of Fatty Acids and Antioxidant Vitamins." *Eur J Cancer* 34:12 (1998): 1852–1856.

Terry, P., P. Lichtenstein, M. Feychting, et al. "Fatty Fish Consumption and Risk of Prostate Cancer." *Lancet* 357:9270 (2001): 1764–1766.

Tsai, W-S, H. Nagawa, S. Kaizaki, et al. "Inhibitory Effects of n-3 Polyunsaturated Fatty Acids on Sigmoid Colon Cancer Transformants." *J Gastroenterol* 33 (1998): 206–212.

Tsujikawa, T., J. Satoh, K. Uda, et al. "Clinical Importance of n-3 Fatty Acid–rich Diet and Nutritional Education for the Maintenance of Remission in Crohn's Disease." *J Gastroenterol* 35:2 (2000): 99–104.

von Schacky, C., P. Angere, W. Kothny, et al. "The Effect of Dietary Omega-3 Fatty Acids on Coronary Atherosclerosis: A Randomized, Double-blind, Placebo-controlled Trial." *Ann Intern Med* 130 (1999): 554–562.

Voskuil, D.W., E.J.M. Feskens, M.B. Katan, et al. "Intake and Sources of Alpha-linolenic Acid in Dutch Elderly Men." *Euro J Clin Nutr* 50:12 (1996): 784–787.

Antioxidants for Disease Prevention

Age-Related Eye Disease Study Research Group (AREDS). "A Randomized, Placebo-controlled, Clinical Trial of High-dose Supplementation with Vitamins C and E, Beta-carotene, and Zinc for Age-related Macular Degeneration and Vision Loss: AREDS Report No. 8." *Arch Ophthalmol* 119 (2001): 1417–1436.

Anonymous. "Antioxidant Vitamins and Zinc for Macular Degeneration." *Med Lett* 45 (2003): 45–46.

Anonymous. "The Effect of Vitamin E and Beta-carotene on the Incidence of Lung Cancer and Other Cancers in Male Smokers. The Alpha-Tocopherol, Beta-carotene Cancer Prevention Study Group." *New Engl J Med* 330:15 (1994): 1029–1035.

Brown, B.G., et al. "Simvastatin and Niacin, Antioxidant Vitamins, or the Combination for the Prevention of Coronary Disease." *New Engl J Med* 345 (2001): 1583–1592.

Freedman, J.E. "Antioxidant versus Lipid-altering Therapy: Some Answers, More Questions." *New Engl J Med* 345 (2001): 1636–1637.

Goldfarb, A.H. "Antioxidants: Role of Supplementation to Prevent Exercise-induced Oxidative Stress (Review)." *Med Sci Sports Exercise* 25:2 (1993): 232–236.

Greenberg, E.R., J.A. Baron, T.D. Tosteson, et al. "A Clinical Trial of Antioxidant Vitamins to Prevent Colorectal Adenoma. Polyp Prevention Study Group." *New Engl J Med* 331:3 (1994): 141–147.

Lee, I.M., et al. "Beta-carotene Supplementation and Incidence of Cancer and Cardiovascular Disease: The Women's Health Study." *J Natl Cancer Inst* 91 (1999): 2102–2106.

Omenn, G.S., et al. "Effects of a Combination of Beta-carotene and Vitamin A on Lung Cancer and Cardiovascular Disease." *New Engl J Med* 334 (1996): 1150–1155.

"Phytochemicals: Drugstore in a Salad?" *Consumer Rep Health* 7 (1995): 133–135.

Rapola, J.M., et al. "Randomized Trial of Alpha-tocopherol and Beta-carotene Supplements on Incidence of Major Coronary Events in Men with Previous Myocardial Infarction." *Lancet* 349 (1997): 1715–1720.

Stampfer, M.J., et al. "Vitamin Consumption and the Risk of Coronary Disease in Women." *New Engl J Med* 328 (1993): 1444–1449.

Tardif, J-C. "Probucol and Multivitamins in the Prevention of Restenosis After Coronary Angioplasty." *New Engl J Med* 337 (1997): 365–372.

The Heart Outcomes Prevention Evaluation Study Investigators. "Vitamin E Supplementation and Cardiovascular Events in High-risk Patients." *New Engl J Med* 342 (2000): 145–153.

Tribble, D.L., et al. "Antioxidant Consumption and Risk of Coronary Heart Disease: Emphasis on Vitamin C, Vitamin E, and Beta-carotene. American Heart Association Science Advisory." *Circulation* 99 (1999): 591-595.

Vivekananthan, D.P., et al. "Use of Antioxidant Vitamins for the Prevention of Cardiovascular Disease: Meta-analysis of Randomized Trials." *Lancet* 361 (2003): 2017–2023.

Trans-Fatty Acids

Ascherio, A., et al. "Trans-fatty Acids and Coronary Heart Disease." *New Engl J Med* 340 (1999): 1994–1998.

Clandinin, M.T., and M.S. Wilke. "Do Trans-fatty Acids Increase the Incidence of Type 2 Diabetes?" *Am J Clin Nutr* 73:6 (2001): 1000–1002.

Hu, F.B., et al. "Dietary Fat Intake and the Risk of Coronary Heart Disease in Women." *New Engl J Med* 337 (1997): 1491–1499.

Hu, F.B., et al. "Diet, Lifestyle, and the Risk of Type 2 Diabetes Mellitus in Women." *New Engl J Med* 343 (2001): 790–797.

Katz, A.M., M.D. "Trans-fatty Acids and Sudden Cardiac Death." *Circulation* 105:6 (2002): 669–671.

Kutubm, K., and F. Sacks. "Trans-Fatty Acid Content of Common Foods." *New Engl J Med* 329 (1993): 1969–1970.

Lichtenstein, A.H., et al. "Hydrogenation Impairs the Hypolipidemic Effect of Corn Oil in Humans." *Arterioscler Thromb* 13:2 (1993): 154–161.

Lichtenstein, A.H., et al. "Effects of Different Forms of Dietary Hydrogenated Fats on Serum Lipoprotein Cholesterol Levels." *New Engl J Med* 340 (1999): 1933–1940.

Lovejoy, J.C. "Dietary Fatty Acids and Insulin Resistance." *Curr Atheroscler Report* 1:3 (1999): 215–220.

Mann, G.V. "Metabolic Consequences of Dietary Trans-fatty Acids." *Lancet* 343:8908 (1994): 1268–1271.

Mensink, R.P., and M.B. Katan. "Effects of Dietary Trans-fatty Acids on High-Density and Low-Density Lipoprotein Cholesterol Levels in Healthy Subjects." *New Engl J Med* 323 (1990): 439–445.

Index

About the Author

Kevin J. Weiland, M.D., F.A.C.P., is a practicing physician, board certified in the specialty of Internal Medicine. He is a graduate of the Sanford School of Medicine of the University of South Dakota and received his Internal Medicine training at the University of Wisconsin Hospital and Clinics in Madison, Wisconsin. He is an associate Professor with the Sanford School of Medicine and is actively involved in numerous non-profit organizations such as the American Cancer Society, American Heart Association, and the American Lung Association. Dr. Weiland is a fellow in the American College of Physicians and is identified as a leader in preventative medicine. He has been recognized with numerous awards for his community service as well as his ongoing work with school nutrition and childhood obesity.

As a columnist, Dr. Weiland writes a monthly article on preventative medicine and has been published in the *Annals of Pharmacology* as well as the State Medical Journal. He is currently the "Supervising Physician" for the documentary movie *Good Meat*.

His experiences with his father while growing up in the funeral business as well as his clinical practice of caring for adults over the years allowed Dr. Weiland to witness first hand, the self-destructive forces of a life style of over-indulgence. His book, *The Dakota Diet*, taps into those experiences and is the driving force for the work in this book. He developed The Dakota Diet as a way to realistically address nutrition and health with his patients. The Dakota Diet is a lifestyle of healthy change, not just a diet found only on the plains of the Dakotas.

Dr. Weiland lives in the Black Hills of South Dakota with his wife, Dr. Laurie Weisensee, and their three children.